Parenting Your
Asperger Child

Parenting Your Asperger Child

INDIVIDUALIZED SOLUTIONS FOR TEACHING
YOUR CHILD PRACTICAL SKILLS

Alan Sohn, Ed.D., and
Cathy Grayson, M.A.

A Perigee Book

A Perigee Book
Published by the Penguin Group
Penguin Group (USA) Inc.
375 Hudson Street, New York, New York 10014, USA
Penguin Group (Canada), 10 Alcorn Avenue, Toronto, Ontario M4V 3B2, Canada
(a division of Pearson Penguin Canada Inc.)
Penguin Books Ltd., 80 Strand, London WC2R 0RL, England
Penguin Group Ireland, 25 St. Stephen's Green, Dublin 2, Ireland (a division of Penguin Books Ltd.)
Penguin Group (Australia), 250 Camberwell Road, Camberwell, Victoria 3124, Australia
(a division of Pearson Australia Group Pty. Ltd.)
Penguin Books India Pvt. Ltd., 11 Community Centre, Panchsheel Park, New Delhi—110 017,
India
Penguin Group (NZ), cnr Airborne and Rosedale Roads, Albany, Auckland 1310, New Zealand
(a division of Pearson New Zealand Ltd.)
Penguin Books (South Africa) (Pty.) Ltd., 24 Sturdee Avenue, Rosebank, Johannesburg 2196,
South Africa
Penguin Books Ltd., Registered Offices: 80 Strand, London WC2R 0RL, England

PRINTING HISTORY
Perigee trade paperback edition / February 2005

PERIGEE is a registered trademark of Penguin Group (USA) Inc.
The "P" design is a trademark belonging to Penguin Group (USA) Inc.

ISBN: 0-399-53070-3

This book has been cataloged by the Library of Congress

PRINTED IN THE UNITED STATES OF AMERICA

10   9   8   7   6   5   4   3   2   1

In memory of my parents, David and Gertrude.
—Alan

For Jon and Josh,
You need to have islands of peace and joy in your life. In my
life, I have been blessed with two: my husband and my son.
—Cathy

ACKNOWLEDGMENTS

From Alan Sohn:

Foremost, I want to thank my wife, Linda. Without her inspiration and prodding, this book would never have been started, let alone completed. She adds credence to the expression: "Behind every good man is an even better woman."

I need to thank both of the Grayson's—Cathy and Jon, Cathy for being my sounding board for ideas; trying them out in her classroom to see if they made any sense. And, also, for being a stickler for details. She took my ideas and gave flesh to them. Thanks to Jon for his willingness to give us entrée into the world of literary agents as well as his frequent critiques of our efforts.

I also need to thank Jessica Lichtenstein and Joelle DelBourgo, our agents, for their advice and direction.

Special thanks to Michael Lutfy, our editor, for his ability to take our ramblings and give them coherence and meaning.

Thanks to my two daughters, Rachel Ferri and Stephanie Cramer, whose professional interest in Asperger's has spurred me on to leave them ideas they can use to help the children with whom they work.

And finally, I must thank the parents and children that I have worked with and continue to see. They have allowed me into their world, shared with me their daily lives, their feelings and their thoughts, allowing me to gain wisdom and compassion so that I might be able to help others in the future.

From Cathy Grayson:

As I look back on my life, I realize I am who I am because of others. My parents, Camillo and Loretta Lupinacci, have believed in me from the day I was born. Their unconditional love has given me the confidence I rely upon in everything that I do. The children and families I have worked with are too numerous to name. The children have made my days interesting and joyful and continually challenge me to think in new ways. The parents of the children I work with have put enormous trust in me, and I have always been humbled by that trust. It has been an honor to work with all of you. Everything I know about Asperger Syndrome I have learned from you.

Writing a book is like giving birth to a baby, and there are certain people whose nurturing makes the book a reality. In this regard I want to thank my agents: To Jessica Lichtenstein, who was excited about this book from the beginning and whose efforts helped this idea grow into a proposal and then a book. Your constant support allowed me to overcome many hurdles. To Joelle DelBourgo who guided me so smoothly through the final stages of the process. To my editor, Michael Lutfy, who edited this book with lightning speed. Thank you for editing my book with such care and for being so very kind to me.

Most important, thanks to my coauthor and friend, Alan Sohn. It has been my pleasure to have worked with you for over twenty-five years. You have deepened my understanding of Asperger Syndrome and have always been there to listen to my questions and concerns. You never let me give up on this book and, yes, you were right!

I have been blessed to have a colleague I can also call a dear friend. Thanks to Becky O'Hara for showing me how to teach social skills the right way, for talking about Asperger Syndrome with me for hours, for sharing life's joys and sorrows, and for providing a daily model of what a true friend looks like. Your friendship has enriched my life.

The best for last, my family. To my son Josh, nothing has ever given me greater joy than being your mom. In wonder, I have watched you grow into a remarkable young man. Thank you for the times when your words of wisdom made the difference. Authors often write, "I could not have written this book without you." In my case that person is my husband Jon. Jon, you patiently agonized over every word with me and treated the book as if it were your own. Without you this book could not have been written. With you as my partner, I've had the joy of being joined with my *bashert*. You are my center, keeping everything that matters in balance. You and Josh complete the very rich tapestry love can be.

CONTENTS

Introduction: Understanding Asperger's Syndrome — 1

1. Cognitive Social Integration Therapy:
Our Approach to Working with the Asperger Child or Teen — 9

2. The Reasons Behind the Behavior — 27

3. Identifying Asperger Subtypes — 47

4. Structure and Predictability:
The Foundation for Change — 63

5. Teaching New Skills — 99

6. Generalization and Sabotage:
How to Make Changes That Last — 137

7. Developing Social Skills: Making and Keeping Friends — 151

8. Crisis Intervention: What to Do During a Crisis — 175

9. Reaching the Final Goal — 197

10. Teaching the Asperger Student:
How to Create an Effective School Program — 205

APPENDICES

A: Characteristics Checklist for Asperger's Syndrome — 229

B: Sohn Grayson Rating Scale for Asperger's Syndrome
and High-Functioning Pervasive Developmental Disorder — 247

C: "How to Play a Game" (Example of a Visual)   252

D: Problem Wheel (Example of a Visual)   254

E: Parent Questionnaire   255

F: End-of-Year Evaluation   257

G: Outline for Evaluation Information for the Asperger Child   259

H: Recommended Social Skills Materials   263

Index   265

About the Authors   273

Understanding Asperger's Syndrome

Before Asperger's syndrome appeared as a high form of autism in 1994 in the American Psychiatric Association's manual, it was no more than a footnote in history. Originally described in the 1940s by Hans Asperger, it was an unclear label even after 1994. It remained uncertain as to which children fell into this category and which did not. Even to this day, the diagnosis still remains very much in the eye of the beholder. There are numerous definitions and characteristics that are applied with varied interpretations.

This is a book about the real world and the Asperger child or teenager. It is not based on theories alone, but on our real-life experiences and the knowledge we have gained from working with children who have been labeled as having Asperger's syndrome, pervasive developmental disorder, semantic pragmatic disorder, high-functioning autistic disorder, a nonverbal learning disability, or some other related disorder. We will use the term *Asperger's* to cover them all.

As painful as it is to accept, it is necessary to understand that the Asperger child or teen is truly different from the typical person. He sees, feels, understands, and acts unlike the rest of the world. He does not understand what is going on around him. This results in miscommunication, misunderstanding, and misperception when he interacts with his peers and those around him, or with society in general. These encounters then cause anxiety and result in considerable rigidity and obsessive-compulsive behaviors.

In order to help the individual with Asperger's syndrome, it is necessary to understand how he interprets the world around him. Those with Asperger's have a neurocognitive disorder that affects many areas of functioning. This includes a difficulty with the basic understanding of the rules of society, especially if they are not explicit. Reading between the lines, understanding various nuances, taking another's perspective, appreciating emotional aspects, comprehending the unspoken rules of a situation, and, most important, understanding social interactions are all difficult to know and/or act upon. As a result, people with Asperger's are prone to making many misinterpretations and inappropriate actions from failing to understand society's rules.

Because the Asperger individual does not understand what is happening in the world, it becomes extremely important for him to keep things just as they are with no changes, additions, or subtractions. Everything needs to go a certain way. Perhaps he should be allowed unlimited computer time. If breakfast comes before getting dressed, it must continue that way. This results in an obsessive-compulsive approach to life. Often, his very first experience with a situation determines how it is supposed to be, and deviation from this experience in the future will not be tolerated. Any changes will cause anxiety, just as not knowing what is going to happen next will also cause anxiety. To reduce his level of anxiety, the Asperger individual creates his own set of rules for everyday functioning to keep things from changing. His rules may be no more than marginally related to what society expects. This leaves him resistant to many of the rules of the world. However, if the overlap with society's rules is greater, his anxiety and his resistance will be less. Those individuals who are able to be more flexible will have less anxiety and will do better.

Since many situations are misunderstood or have a different set of operating rules, the Asperger individual may want to withdraw or avoid them. Escape into fantasy is often a common response. When he cannot withdraw or escape, his anxiety level will increase to the point of upset. If escape is not possible, he will often become more rigid and attempt to control people and events. By narrowing the events, situations, experiences, people, foods, or activities that he comes in contact with, he can reduce the possibility for upset.

There are cognitive trade-offs for the Asperger individual. He usually has an excellent rote memory for facts since they do not require interpretation. Visual processing of information is also well developed, which leads to a high level of skill with word and number recognition. Abstractions and interpretations are more difficult, as are conditions that are subtle, implied, or vague, and this can apply to even the smallest of situations.

The Six Characteristics of Asperger's Syndrome

Each of the following six traits are outlined in detail in the checklist in appendix A, which we recommend you complete after reading this introduction. Only a brief explanation will be provided here.

1. Difficulty with Reciprocal Social Interactions

Those with Asperger's syndrome display varying difficulties when interacting with others. Some children and adolescents have no desire to interact, while others simply do not know how. More specifically, they do not comprehend the give-and-take nature of social interactions. They may want to lecture you about the *Titanic* or they may leave the room in the midst of playing with another child. They do not comprehend the verbal and nonverbal cues used to further our understanding in typical social interactions. These include eye contact, facial expressions, body language, conversational turn-taking, perspective taking, and matching conversational and nonverbal responses to the interaction.

2. Impairments in Language Skills

Those with Asperger's syndrome have very specific problems with language, especially with *pragmatic* use of language, which is the social aspect. That is, they see language as a way to share facts and information (especially about special interests), not as a way to share thoughts, feelings, and emotions. The child will display difficulty in many areas of a conversation—processing verbal information, initiation, maintenance, ending, topic appropriateness, sustaining attention, and turn taking. The child's *prosody* (pitch, stress, rhythm, or melody of speech) can also be impaired. Conversations may often appear scripted or ritualistic. That is, it may be dialogue from a TV show or a movie. They may also have difficulty problem solving, analyzing or synthesizing information, and understanding language beyond the literal level.

3. Narrow Range of Interests and Insistence on Set Routines

Due to the an Asperger child's anxiety, his interactions will be ruled by rigidity, obsessions, and *perseverations* (repetitious behaviors or language) transitions and changes can cause. Generally, he will have few interests, but those interests will often dominate. The need for structure and routine will be most important. He may develop his own rules to live by that barely coincide with the rest of society.

4. Motor Clumsiness

Many individuals with Asperger's syndrome have difficulty with both gross and fine motor skills. The difficulty is often not just the task itself, but the motor planning involved in completing the task. Typical difficulties include handwriting, riding a bike, and ball skills.

5. Cognitive Issues

Mindblindness, or the inability to make inferences about what another person is thinking, is a core disability for those with Asperger's syndrome. Because of this, they have difficulty empathizing with others, and will often say what they think without considering another's feelings. The child will often assume that everyone is thinking the same thing he is. For him, the world exists not in shades of gray, but only in black and white. This rigidity in thought (lack of cognitive flexibility) interferes with problem solving, mental planning, impulse control, flexibility in thoughts and actions, and the ability to stay focused on a task until completion. The rigidity also makes it difficult for an Asperger child to engage in imaginative play. His interest in play materials, themes, and choices will be narrow, and he will attempt to control the play situation.

6. Sensory Sensitivities

Many Asperger children have sensory issues. These can occur in one or all of the senses (sight, sound, smell, touch, or taste). The degree of difficulty varies from one individual to another. Most frequently, the child will perceive ordinary sensations as quite intense or may even be underreactive to a sensation. Often, the challenge in this area will be to determine if the child's response to a sensation is actually a sensory reaction or if it is a learned behavior, driven mainly by rigidity and anxiety.

Understanding This Book

To be able to help an Asperger child or teen, you must learn to think as he does. Problems arise not only from his neurological deficits, but also from professionals who don't fully understand Asperger's or who have mistakenly diagnosed another disorder. As a result, parents and professionals are not adequately preparing these children to survive in the real world. They are using stickers and points to obtain good behavior. They prompt, but do not teach. They do not comprehend that real-life survival skills are needed to replace the child's inappropriate behavior. They do not comprehend that skills need to be developed for self-calming, managing stress, coping with disappointments, dealing with surprises, and doing things differently. These skills, and many others, are necessary to help your Asperger child fit into society.

Over the years, we have witnessed all kinds of tantrums. We know what it is to "walk on eggshells" to avoid upsetting your child. We understand the pain in seeing your child sitting home alone while other children are playing outside. From these situations, we have discovered what can help, what works and what doesn't.

As we worked with these children, we discovered the key to helping them. Most Asperger children have a profound interest in words. Language helps all of us to understand what is going on in our lives and allows us to develop the strategies to deal with these issues. Your Asperger child probably does not know how to use his language to understand and solve problems, but we can teach him how. This approach can be especially powerful for those who are intellectually gifted, but that is not a requirement. However, those children who do not have at least average language and intellectual ability will have more difficulty understanding the language-based solutions that form the basis of our program.

We call our approach Cognitive Social Integration Therapy (CSIT). It is a practical, hands-on approach. It's cognitive because we believe behavioral changes occur through understanding and the thinking processes, not through simple rewards and punishments. Our goal is to teach the skills your child is lacking to help him function in society. Through step-by-step practice, we help him understand why his behavior is a problem and specifically what he has to do differently to change it. To do this, you, as well as others, must change the way you interact with your child. Too often, people wait until something goes wrong and then try to do something about it. This is a completely backward approach for an Asperger individual. Prevention is the key. Anticipate problems, plan for them, and implement your plan before a problem arises.

But simply stopping undesirable behaviors is not sufficient. You need to teach replacement skills for that behavior. You need to explain how the world operates, why certain things are done, then convince your Asperger child why these ideas are better than his own. After all, your child acts the way he does because he has a different view of the world than the rest of us.

CSIT, therefore, has a social component in the broadest sense. Almost everything your child does requires social skills because other people are almost always involved in every facet of his life. Cooperating with others instead of trying to control situations is a social skill. Being flexible instead of rigid in solving a problem is also a social skill. Dealing with anxiety-producing problems instead of avoiding them is a social skill. CSIT uses language to help your child deal with these social and behavioral encounters, which ultimately will improve his understanding of the world and help him to develop the social skills needed to fit in with society as a productive and independent citizen.

But we don't stop with improvement. We want more than that. We want growth. This can only come when your child's new skills can be applied to other settings. We teach you how to intentionally cause problems to strengthen these skills and make them a part of your child's life. We even teach you how to learn something from a crisis. This goes against some conventional therapies, which focus mainly on survival. We do that, but much more. We teach you how to help your child to thrive and to grow.

To help you pinpoint specific goals, and to thoroughly familiarize yourself with Asperger's and your child's particular version of it, you should complete the Characteristics Checklist and the Sohn Grayson Rating Scale found in appendices A and B. We encourage you to copy these tools and share them with others who are involved in caring for your child—teachers, therapists, relatives, caregivers, and so on. When completing the checklist, check off all the characteristics that apply to your child. Use the examples that are given as illustrations. Your child may display the same behavior or his own particular variation. In any case, once you have completed the checklist, do the same for the Sohn Grayson Rating Scale. Match the areas your child experiences the biggest difficulties with from the rating scale with the same areas on the checklist. You will now have a detailed explanation of each problem area. These will be the areas that need further skill development by whoever will be working with your child. As you learn more of the details of CSIT, these two instruments will help you to tailor our program to fit the needs of your child.

1

Cognitive Social Integration Therapy

OUR APPROACH TO WORKING WITH
THE ASPERGER CHILD OR TEEN

"I Can See Clearly Now"

Though children with Asperger's syndrome display similar characteristics, we know from experience that every child arrives with his or her own special "twist" on Asperger's, and you must look beyond the obvious. In the Asperger world, things are not always as they appear, and even the smallest deviations need to be investigated. Even after many years of working with ritualistic behavior, we are always discovering new ones.

For example, Noah, a six-year-old with Asperger's, had been successfully taking the district van to school for the first month of school. An administrative transportation problem arose with the van service and the responsibility for getting Noah to school fell to his parents.

This change allowed us to become aware of a particular ritual Noah engaged in. As soon as he entered his parents' car he would strip off his clothes and refuse to dress until they arrived at their destination and he would be leaving the car. After gathering more information and questioning Noah's parents we discovered this behavior had been taking place since Noah was three and would occur even when their destination was only five minutes away. In addition, if they were running errands and had a number of stops, this was repeated at each stop. "It's a real problem in the winter," his dad said. "We try to bring a quilt or a blanket so he won't be so cold." Obviously, this problem needed to be addressed immediately.

Although his parents were concerned and inconvenienced by his behavior, they saw no way out; they believed their son had sensory sensitivities and this was one of its manifestations. We asked them, If this really was a sensory issue, wouldn't Noah do this anytime he was in a car? They agreed and said he also did this with his grandparents, the only other people he rode with. What about the school van, we asked, why wasn't he removing his clothes when the van was taking him to school? This thought had not occurred to Noah's parents. They had become so accustomed to his behavior that it no longer seemed unusual or a problem that needed to be changed. Perhaps his stripping had initially been a response to a sensory sensitivity, but over time it had become a habit.

Both Noah and his parents needed to see this situation in a new way: as a problem we were going to solve. The solution turned out to be relatively easy and painless. Noah and I created a social story (a technique described in chapter 8) that discussed appropriate dress when in a car or van. Initially, Noah was rewarded for this behavior. Since Noah was a "rule boy" (see chapter 3), the social story gave him the rules, and, thus, the behavior he needed to display.

Why hadn't Noah's parents done something before this time? How long had they allowed this situation to continue? Noah's parents reacted the same way many parents do when faced with a similar dilemma— maybe it is best to leave the problem alone. After all, who is harmed by it? Any attempt to change behaviors often results in prolonged tantrums, so let's leave well enough alone. Little do they realize this is one of many obsessions that will need to be dealt with in the future, because obsessions, anxiety, rigidity, and tantrums only grow as the child gets older.

You cannot indulge your Asperger child's quirks or peculiar behaviors, allowing him to obsess on the weather or modes of transportation. You cannot allow him to kiss other students whom he likes. Your job is to help your child learn to cope with the demands of society, and learn how the world operates. If your child cannot fit into society to some degree, he will not be able to fully realize the many strengths and gifts he possesses. Each problem you encounter provides an opportunity to help the individual with Asperger's to fit into society a little better, and that should always be your goal. Never be afraid to seize those opportunities.

Defenders of Reality

When parents seek help for their child, they encounter varied opinions—he'll outgrow it, leave him alone, it's no big deal, he just wants attention, and so on. Many professionals try to work with the Asperger child as if his disorder is like other developmental disorders, but it is quite different. In most cases, there is a great misunderstanding by many people of the needs of these special individuals.

Diagnosis Can Be Difficult

For the inexperienced, recognizing the six defining characteristics of Asperger's as outlined in the introduction can be difficult, and misdiagnoses are quite common. This is further complicated by the fact that an Asperger child or teen has many of the same characteristics found in other disorders. These various characteristics are often misinterpreted, overlooked, underemphasized, or overemphasized. As a result, a child may receive many different diagnoses over time or from different professionals.

For example, if a child with Asperger's demonstrates a high degree of attention deficit hyperactivity disorder (ADHD), that might be the only diagnosis he receives. However, this is a common characteristic of Asperger children. The same holds true if obsessive or compulsive behaviors are displayed—the child gets labeled with obsessive-compulsive disorder (OCD) instead of Asperger's. The following traits are also commonly seen in those with Asperger's syndrome in varying degrees. However, just because these traits are there, it doesn't mean that the child should be diagnosed differently; these traits should be noted as significant features of Asperger's:

- Anxiety

- Hyperlexia (advanced word recognition skills)

- Sensory difficulties

- Motor deficits

- Difficulty with pragmatic language skills

- Social skills deficits

- Oppositional defiant disorder (ODD)

As mentioned, professionals who do not have much experience with Asperger's have a hard time identifying the defining characteristics. For example, social skill deficits may be noted by a professional, but then they are often downplayed because the child or adolescent appears to be having appropriate conversations with others or seems to be interested in other people. But with an Asperger child, the conversations are not generally reciprocal, so the child must be carefully observed to see whether or not there is true back-and-forth interaction. Also, many Asperger children have an interest in others, but you need to clarify if the objects of their interest are age appropriate. Do they interact with peers in an age-appropriate fashion? Can they maintain friendships over a period of time or do they end as the novelty wears off? These are the types of observations and questions that must be asked in order to ensure a proper diagnosis.

Another example of an overlooked area is the narrow routines or rituals that are supposed to be present. This does not always manifest as obsessive-compulsive behavior in the typical sense, such as repeated handwashing or neatness, but rather in the insistence on the need for rules about many issues and situations. These children may not throw tantrums over their need for rules, but may require them just as much as the person who has a meltdown when a rule is violated. In essence, there is no single profile of the typical Asperger individual. They are not all the same, as you will see in later chapters.

Because of these subtleties and nuances, the single most important consideration in diagnosis is that the person making the initial diagnosis be familiar with autistic spectrum disorders—in particular, Asperger's syndrome. They should have previously diagnosed numerous children. To make a proper, initial diagnosis requires the following:

1. You (both parents) and your child should have sessions with a psychologist where your child is carefully observed to see how he responds in various situations. This is done through play or talk sessions in the psychologist's office and by discussions with both parents. The psychologist may ask you to complete checklists or questionnaires to gain a better understanding of the child's behaviors at home and/or school. If the child is in school, the psychologist may call the child's teacher or ask her to complete additional checklists. The checklists or questionnaires used should be ones that are appropriate for individuals with Asperger's syndrome. It is important to determine the IQ level of your child as well. An average or above-average IQ is necessary for a diagnosis of Asperger's.

2. The child should see a neurologist or developmental pediatrician (again, someone familiar with autistic spectrum disorders) for a thorough neurological exam to rule out other medical conditions and to assess the need for medication. The physician may suggest additional medical testing (blood, urine, fragile X, hearing).

3. It is important to include a speech and language evaluation, as those with Asperger's syndrome will display impairments in the pragmatics and semantics of language, despite having adequate receptive and expressive language. This will also serve to make parents aware of any unusual language patterns the child displays that will interfere in later social situations. Again, these oddities may not be recognized if the evaluator is not familiar with Asperger's syndrome.

4. Finally, an evaluation by an occupational therapist familiar with sensory integration difficulties may provide additional and valuable information.

Now that you have a diagnosis, the first thing most likely on your mind is what to do about it. Professionals and books often offer advice that is vague and overly general, as if everyone already knows exactly what to do. Nothing could be further from the truth. Those with Asperger's require a very specific and unique approach, a practical, step-by-step approach that tells you how to make the changes that are necessary.

Many interventions employ a traditional "rewards and consequences" approach, which is rarely effective because it focuses on what happens after the event you want to change has already occurred. The approach we advocate here is proactive so that you can prevent problems or at least reduce their frequency and intensity. If you are discussing a problem before it has occurred, there is less emotion since nothing has gone wrong.

You are also preparing your child for a change in his routine or a new way of doing something. Advanced warnings/preparations are the single most important technique to use, and they must occur before an event. While this sounds easy, it is difficult only because it is a new way to think about problems and their solutions. Most people think about a solution after the problem has occurred; they are usually thinking about a consequence only, not a replacement behavior. Those with Asperger's rarely learn something from a consequence; therefore, it does not prevent them from repeating the undesirable behavior. Sure, they are upset with the consequence, but that should never be the goal of any intervention. We don't just want empty promises about the next time. The real goal is always behavior change. We want things to go better.

It is important to realize that Asperger children have limited ability to problem solve and are not able to observe what they are doing. So, they are not always embarrassed by what they say or do. They do not experience internal conflict as we might. They find it difficult to self-correct, self-evaluate, or self-monitor. In other words, they can't see that their behavior is wrong or is causing a problem. They are not upset about being inappropriate. They have a limited set of skills to use when things go wrong and so they use them in all situations. If being angry and hitting is used in some settings, it will be used in many situations; the same for crying or yelling. If controlling their environment is their solution of choice, it will be used whenever a problem occurs. They cannot easily make behavioral choices or evaluate a situation. It is not that they do not think of others. They *can't*. It's not as if they want to be in charge. They *must* be. Therefore, you must be the one to help them understand the way the world works and how they must learn to fit in. You must be the "defender of reality."

Cognitive Social Integration Therapy

In order to understand how the world works, the Asperger individual needs a comprehensive plan; that plan is Cognitive Social Integration Therapy (CSIT). CSIT is a comprehensive treatment approach we have developed to treat those with Asperger's syndrome. The approach is to be used by all of the people (psychiatrists, psychologists, counselors, teachers, speech and language therapists, occupational therapists, and, of course, parents) who are involved with the Asperger child in all of the environments (therapy sessions, classroom, at home) he inhabits. It is critical that those using it understand what CSIT is and how to use it effectively.

What Is Cognitive Social Integration Therapy?

CSIT recognizes the primary deficit of Asperger's syndrome is an inability to understand societal rules and engage in reciprocal (back-and-forth, give-and-take, etc.) social interactions. Because of their neurological deficits, Asperger children and teens fail to understand their own thoughts and feelings, as well as those of others. In addition, they are not able to problem solve effectively. Their difficulties with social understanding and expression, perspective taking, and problem solving influence all aspects of their lives and, in particular, significantly compromise their ability to converse. Furthermore, this lack of understanding, which results in frequent feelings of confusion regarding how the world works, causes them to be in a near constant state of anxiety. The resulting anxiety leads to the development of the many secondary characteristics (rigidity, repetitive behavior, obsessive-compulsive behavior, being rule bound, insistence on sameness, narrow interests) displayed by those with Asperger's syndrome.

Unlike other approaches used to treat those with Asperger's syndrome, the role of anxiety is not overlooked in CSIT and is addressed in both its prevention and its intervention strategies. Based on our experience, we regard the child or teen with Asperger's syndrome as a thinking person who has thoughts and feelings. Though these feelings may be atypical, their presence must be addressed. The child's thoughts and feelings must be acknowledged and modified to allow him to function more productively and without constant anxiety. His ability to discuss the Greek language in extraordinary detail may soothe his anxiety, but will eventually turn off his peers. Alternative ways must be provided to decrease the Asperger child's anxiety.

We believe in a prevention model, creating environments that reduce anxiety, introducing skills that will prevent anxiety when changes occur, and allowing the child to interact more effectively by teaching new skills and expanding repertoires. Because we recognize that not all skills can be taught, and not all anxiety can be avoided, intervention and crisis strategies to use at these times are also incorporated.

In summary, three distinct areas are developed through CSIT:

1. Prevention strategies to increase understanding and avoid difficulties when change occurs

2. Generalization strategies and the expansion of existing repertoires through planned change (sabotage)

3. Crisis intervention strategies to help the child regain control when problems occur, combined with the teaching of more effective responses for the future

How Is CSIT Used?

Our approach is based on developing new skills, not on simple redirection or prompting. It is a prevention/proactive model, not a reaction/

consequence model. We have found that a direct instruction model provides the most effective treatment. Areas of need are identified (social skills, perspective taking, conversational skills, special interests, obsessive-compulsive behaviors, and rigidity/routines) and skills are taught both verbally and visually, using rehearsal, role playing, and guided practice. Treatment focuses on not only what to do, but how to do it. Examples are given, not simply explanations. Each skill is broken down into small steps (task analysis) and taught in a structured format. It is assumed the child lacks the necessary skills and/or does not recognize that skills from previous experiences may apply to a new situation; therefore, all aspects must be taught. Along with systematic and direct instruction of skills, the following goals make up the core components of CSIT.

The Seven Core Components of CSIT

Our purpose is to foster a true understanding of the world of those living with Asperger's syndrome. There is a profound difference between knowing about a problem and understanding it. Our goal is *understanding*. In order to accomplish this, we've developed seven core components of CSIT that will be discussed throughout this book.

Understanding Why He Acts the Way He Does— The Reasons Behind the Behavior

One day in late March, Zack, a ten-year-old, entered the library with his mother and easily responded to the librarian's greeting. She then asked him a question about one of the books he was returning. Zack had been attending weekly story time since he was four. A voracious reader, he borrowed his limit of books each week from the library. He and his mother were a familiar sight there. Some of the staff, and this librarian in particular, had taken the time to understand Zack and Asperger's syndrome. He especially liked this librarian because he enjoyed listening to her stories and, on a few occasions, she had reserved books about electricity (his special interest) for him. After the conversation went back and forth twice, Zack asked the librarian an inappropriate and hurtful question. Because of her prior experience with Zack, she responded firmly and appropriately. When he left the library, his mother immediately took Zack aside to provide him with an understanding of what had happened. He had been working on conversational skills and his behavior surprised her. She began by asking him about the question he had asked and exploring his understanding of it. Before she had gone very far, he said to her, "I know it was mean, but we learned the rule that conversations go back and forth. I didn't know what to say, so I said that to keep the conversation going."

On the surface, or to those not experienced with the Asperger's, Zack's behavior appeared rude. For Zack, it was a way to follow the rules he had been taught and to converse with someone he genuinely liked. While this example occurred at the library, it could have been at the mall, a party, at school, or anywhere where the individual had to interact with another without the necessary script. Our experience tells us preparation is as important as the actual intervention. Proper preparation will determine the success of your interventions.

We believe you must have a clear understanding of the motivation behind the child's behaviors before intervening. You must carefully look "behind the behavior," because what often appears to be the reason for a particular behavior is no more than an inaccurate assumption. With CSIT you are trying to identify the true function of the behavior—what does the child think she is trying to accomplish? Our experience with Asperger's tells us her behavior is usually a function of one or more of the following:

- A need to engage in or continue a preferred activity, often an obsessive action or fantasy—*"I can't come to the dinner table until I count all my books."*

- A need to avoid/escape a nonpreferred activity—*"I can't go to the birthday party, I might throw up"* (in this case throwing up is simply an excuse, not a real fear).

- A violation of a rule or ritual—*"I can't eat breakfast today, there's no orange juice."*

• A misunderstanding/misinterpretation of another's action—*"No! John didn't push me by accident when we were playing basketball. It was on purpose."*

• A need to control a situation—*"We have to go to Grandma's house on Route 5, we always go that way."*

• A need for immediate gratification—*"I don't care if the TV is broken, I have to watch it now."*

• A transition from one activity to another—*"It's hard for me to change from reading to math."*

• Internal issues (sensory, inattention, oppositional tendency, psychiatric issues)—*"I can't get my hair cut, the hair place is too noisy."*

Before you address an issue, know the issue you plan to address. Again, our experience tells us preparation is as important as the actual intervention. Proper preparation will determine the success of your interventions.

Designing Strategies Based on Asperger Subtypes

Tommy, a six-year-old, wanted to be in charge of every situation. When asked about this, he replied that he wanted to be king. Since he was a "logic boy," he was told that there is no royalty in the United States, just a president. But he couldn't be that either, because you had to be at least thirty-five years old. Finally, it was pointed out that a six-year-old really can't be in charge of anyone else. They must listen to their teachers and their parents.

Emma, an eight-year-old, was easily upset by anything different that occurred in her life. If it was picture day at school, she was upset. If she received a warning in school about her behavior, she was upset. If the family went to a restaurant she didn't like, she was upset. Just about everything upset her. Every attempt to provide reasons and explanations for her, to prepare her, or to have her agree to a solution was not successful. She was too anxious to comply. All of these interventions were a mismatch in helping someone with anxiety to cope. Anxiety-reducing techniques would have been much more appropriate.

It is imperative for your interventions to be customized to fit the child's cognitive ability, language skills, and personality type. If you have not already done so, complete both the Characteristics Checklist and the Sohn Grayson Rating Scale found in appendices A and B. Not all children with Asperger's are the same. Chapter 3 will describe the different subtypes and how to tailor interventions to their needs. In the above example, Tommy needs logic to understand how things make sense. Rational and detailed clarifications give him the logical explanations he needs. Emma, on the other hand, is driven by anxiety, so anxiety-reduction techniques, rather than logic-based interventions, will be more effective. Without understanding the subtype, you cannot develop an effective behavior plan for change.

Working with Structure and Predictability— The Foundation for Change

Ethan, a fourteen-year-old, was having great difficulty at home. Almost all requests from his parents, whether simple (get your coat) or more involved (it's time for homework), were met with refusal. His parents were beginning to avoid placing any demands on him, even in areas where he had been successful. The resulting tantrums were just too big a price to pay. Their concern led them to ask for help, and we began to structure his home life. A daily schedule was created, a list of rules was developed, appropriate behaviors were modeled and practiced, and rewards/consequences were developed that made use of preferred versus nonpreferred activities as a natural consequence. By the end of the second week, his parents reported his behavior was steadily improving. Upon praising him for his hard work and good behavior, he replied, "I like my house now. I know what to do."

Take a moment to imagine the following. You don't understand the world around you. You don't know what people want. You often feel anxious, confused, and worried. You find if you create your own world, with your own rules and routines, you are less anxious and not so confused. Unfortunately, your rules (barking when noises are too loud, introducing yourself as Batman, only eating foods of a certain color) clash with those of the world around you. The people you are involved with attempt to prevent you from following your rules and routines, without providing you with adequate alternatives. When they interrupt your rules and routines, it feels as if they are being unfair, breaking the rules and causing your anxiety to return. In response, you act out, withdraw, or create more and more rules and routines.

The model we have developed sets the stage for intervention by providing the child or teen with a consistent and structured environment. We relieve anxiety, begin to answer the question, "What's going on?" and present alternative ways of responding.

Becoming a Sphere of Influence

There are two statements my students make about me that I consider the highest form of praise. The first is, "Go ask Mrs. Grayson about your problem. Didn't you know she is a problem solver?" The second is, "You better listen to her. She means what she says."

Our goal for those working with Asperger's is to help them become a sphere of influence—individuals who can exert influence over the child's view of and interactions with the world. Your ability to achieve this will determine your success in teaching replacement skills. Our experience has taught us you must learn to anticipate problems before they occur. In so doing, your control of the situation assists the Asperger child in gaining/maintaining his own control. You must anticipate problems before they occur.

Making Changes That Last—Generalization and Sabotage

Sara, a twelve-year-old, visited Longwood Gardens with her family to enjoy the recently arrived spring weather. They passed other families and groups also enjoying the extensive greenhouse, conservatory, and gardens. After passing a group of elderly women on a tour, Sara turned to her mother and said, "Mom, those ladies were really, really old, but I know that's something I have to keep in my head. You know, like I can't tell Uncle Bill his teeth are yellow."

Eric, a seven-year-old, entered the classroom with a big smile on his face. "Mrs. Grayson, I was flexible this morning. I was flexible. My mom told me I was great." I replied, "That's super, Eric. What did you do?" "I put my shoes on before I had breakfast, rather than after. You know I always did it that way for a long time."

Over time, we have realized the power of language when working with Asperger's. Language used in a concrete, predictable manner will increase comprehension. As comprehension increases, so does compliance, and your child's anxiety will begin to decrease. With CSIT, language creates a road map of understanding—a means to negotiate unfamiliar territory. We consistently use a variety of key words and phrases to help those with Asperger's syndrome internalize new ways of thinking and responding to confusing or challenging situations. A brief list of key phrases includes:

- *In your head* (thoughts about others you may not share)

- *Problems and solutions* (you have a problem and I can help you solve it)

- *Just do it* (this request is not a choice, but a rule to be followed quickly)

- *Drop the subject* (a conversation is concluded immediately)

- *Stretching the topic* (attempts to make something off topic appear on topic)

The child's internalization of phrases like these fosters generalization. If you are successful, you will see that the language cues, phrases, and concepts you introduce will change as they generalize from adult-directed cues to prompted cues to child-directed cues. With our model you are provided with a structure of how to develop and effectively use language cues, as well as how to present concepts, such as flexibility.

In our work with Asperger children and teens, we have found that programming generalization and using planned sabotage to teach flexibility is crucial. Sabotage is our way of introducing change in a controlled manner to maximize the chances of the child's success. We have learned that changes in behavior come from a need, and sabotage creates a need for the child to engage in a behavior we have previously taught. By using consistent language, supplying rules to relieve anxiety, and providing a road map of expected behavior, we introduce stability into their confused world. The rules answer the question, "What do I do?" by letting them know what they can and cannot do. Combined with demonstrations of "how to do it," CSIT allows you to expand the child's repertoire of coping.

In the example earlier in this chapter, Noah's car behavior is a perfect illustration of this. Noah's perception of riding in a car included the removal of all his clothes. Initially, the idea of riding in a car and staying dressed was presented as a social story. However, this was not enough—it had to become a rule to provide the necessary structure. A few months later, we saw how very important this was. I was going through Noah's desk to check his handwriting book. When he saw me removing items from his desk he said, "Mrs. Grayson, don't take my car story. If you do I won't know what to do." At this point, undressing in the car was no longer an issue—for the past few weeks we had not even read the story! However, the story's power and influence were still apparent.

Surviving a Crisis and Learning from It

"I hate you. I hate this bowling alley. I hate birthday parties," Andrew, a nine-year-old, screamed while being removed from his friend's birthday party. His father calmly led him to a private and quiet location and repeated the following: "You are having a problem and I will help you solve it. As soon as you stop screaming we can work on solving your problem. You have a problem and I am a problem solver."

No matter how much effort is put into prevention and skills training, crisis situations will occur. Our crisis intervention strategies are used to stop inappropriate behaviors and teach more appropriate responses for the future. In a crisis, the first step is to help the child to calm down. Nothing can be accomplished while someone is screaming, hitting, crying, or being destructive. Your demeanor and language are crucial during this period. Once the child is calm, you can then ask him to comply with a simple request. If he is able to do this, you have successfully completed step one, getting through the tantrum phase. However, it is critical for this to be followed by step two: problem solving. Problem solving represents the part of a crisis where learning for the future can occur. During this phase you present and teach alternative or new behaviors, which can be used in place of the inappropriate behaviors the child has been using.

Reaching the Final Goal—I'm Okay, You're Okay

"We met when I was in second grade. I was in trouble and Dr. Sohn came. He was there to help me solve my problems. This is the cause and effect. I am mad. I take it out on the teachers. I get in trouble. Dr. Sohn comes and reasons it out. Then my troubles are over," Kevin, age eight, reported.

Joey, a ten-year-old, had to control everything in his life. Every person in his life had to follow the rules he created, and there were plenty of them. You couldn't call him Joseph, it was always Joe or Joey. He had to sit on his legs. His feet were not allowed to touch the floor. If you made him do something he did not like, he would scream and threaten to fire you or eat you up. After intervening, these issues were resolved: You could call him by any name; however, he'd calmly say he preferred Joe. He put his feet on the floor, not because he liked it, but because it was the right way for fifth graders to sit. And if you had him do something he didn't like, he'd attempt to compromise with you to reach an amicable settlement.

It is never enough just to get by and survive day-to-day. You want your child to have feelings of control and competence over his environment; to be more in line with society's rules; to be less rigid, which reduces anxiety; to expand his narrow repertoire of interests; to know how to cooperate and comply with others' rules; and to act with increasing independence to be the best he can be. In essence, to be okay. At the same time, you need to feel everything is not a battle anymore. You, too, need to be okay. And life becomes a more cooperative adventure for all.

Now that you understand the philosophy of our intervention approach to Asperger's syndrome, you are ready to learn about the reasons behind the behaviors the child or teen is displaying. In the next chapter you will learn the answers to the questions: What is the function of a behavior? What roles do anxiety and obsessive-compulsive behaviors play? and How can preferred activities be used as a reinforcer for completing nonpreferred activities? Our focus is on understanding behaviors and the motivations that sustain them. In so doing, you will be able to select, prioritize, and develop appropriate goals.

2

The Reasons Behind the Behavior

Twelve-year-old Steven would never throw anything away, nor would he allow anyone else to discard anything. When his parents purchased a new sofa, he insisted that they keep the old one, along with the box it came in. He always brought home his trash from his school lunch, unable to throw it into the school trash can. He could not part with old clothing, either, even if it was worn out or no longer fit.

Eventually Steven needed new lenses for his eyeglasses because he could no longer see well, but he refused to have them changed. His parents actually did not see any connection between this problem and Steven's refusal to part with other things. It took some discussion before they realized all of these behavioral issues were related to the same thing: Steven's resistance to change. He never wanted anything to change, and throwing something out was about as permanent a change as you could make. There was no way he would allow his lenses to be changed without throwing a tantrum. "I can see fine out of my old ones. They're just dirty," he would scream.

The first thing we did was to gather information about other difficulties Steven had with change to determine the reasons behind his behavior. This led to a discussion about the similarity of many of Steven's sources of upset. By pointing out how many other events were similar, Steven was able to see the connection between his glasses and everything else that he insisted on saving, and it became clear to everyone that even the smallest change in this pattern would be a problem. He had an obsession. No amount of reward, cajoling, or threatening was going to change it.

We needed to help him develop the skills to cope with change, and that included getting rid of things. We also had to decide what the first issue to change would be. Sometimes we don't start with the very first issue we encounter because it is a goal too difficult to attain at first. Not all goals are equally difficult for your child. So we try to find a similar goal that may be easier to start with. Very soon after we began, Steven was not only able to get new glasses, but he allowed his parents to throw away the sofa and the carton it came in. We achieved what we wanted by creating a list of goals for him to achieve. We started with a very small goal to desensitize him to the change that occurs when getting rid of things. We started with very small items, gradually moving on to items of greater importance. We added forced choices in which he had to choose one thing or another to discard, and we didn't allow any whining or crying to deter us from our goal. How we achieved these goals will be clear as you read through this book.

Many parents try to change their child's behavior in a moment of desperation, without giving thought as to *why* the behavior is occurring. This is known as the *function of the behavior* and refers to the reason behind the action. General, all-purpose, hit-or-miss strategies are often used that don't address the specific Asperger-caused deficit. To yell, coax, threaten, or promise rewards are not effective strategies. They do not teach new skills that are necessary for change. You need to understand what your child or teenager is thinking, how he interprets what is going on, and how his deficits cause problems before you can begin any intervention strategy. Do not rush into action until you have collected enough information and analyzed what is going on. If you do not know the reasons behind the behavior, you may very likely do the wrong thing. If you know what is going on, you can help things go better.

Realizing that your child will not be a good observer of his behavior is your first step. The Asperger child often does not know what to do in a situation. He does not know the appropriate behavior because he doesn't understand how the world works. Or, if he knows a better solution, he cannot use it because he becomes "stuck."

Not knowing what to do, or being unable to do what is appropriate, results in anxiety that leads to additional ineffective and inappropriate actions. An Asperger behavior is usually a result of this anxiety, which leads to difficulty moving on and letting go of an issue and "getting stuck" on something. This is *rigidity*, and it is the most common reason for behavioral problems. See the sidebar for a list of reasons for rigidity. You must deal with rigidity and replace it with *flexibility* early on in your plan to help your child. Flexibility is a skill that can be taught, and you will make this a major part of your efforts to help your child.

REASONS FOR RIGIDITY

1. Lack of knowledge about how something is done. By not knowing how the world works with regard to specific situations and events, the child will act inappropriately instead.

2. The need to avoid or escape from a nonpreferred activity, often something difficult or undesirable. Often, if your child cannot be perfect, she does not want to engage in an activity.

3. The need to engage in or continue a preferred activity, usually an obsessive action or fantasy.

4. A violation of a rule or ritual—changing something from the way it is supposed to be. Someone is violating a rule and this is unacceptable to the child.

5. Anxiety about a current or upcoming event, no matter how trivial it might appear to you.

6. A misunderstanding or misinterpretation of another's action.

7. The need to control a situation.

8. Immediate gratification of a need.

9. Transitioning from one activity to another. This is usually a problem because it may mean ending an activity before he is finished with it.

10. Other internal issues, such as sensory, inattention (ADHD), oppositional tendency (ODD), or other psychiatric issues may also be causes of behavior.

Note: Attention-getting is very rarely seen. It should not be considered as a reason for rigidity until all of the above reasons have been considered and eliminated.

Understanding your child involves knowing the Asperger characteristics discussed earlier and how they manifest themselves in everyday behaviors. How does your child or adolescent see the world, think about matters, and react to what is going on around him? The following reasons will help you understand "why he acts the way he does."

Not Understanding How the World Works

Your Asperger child has a neurocognitive disorder that affects many areas of functioning. This includes a difficulty with the basic understanding of the rules of society, especially if they are not obvious. Life has many of these rules. Some are written, some are spoken, and some are learned through observation and intuition. Your child only knows what has been directly taught to him through books, movies, TV shows, the Internet, and explicit instructions. He is not able to sit in a room, observe what is happening, and understand social cues, implied directions, or how to "read between the lines," and as he is growing up, he does not learn how to do this. Instead, he learns facts. He does not "take in" what is happening around him that involves the rest of the world, only what directly impacts him.

Many of the conversations he has had have generally been about knowledge and facts, not about feelings, opinions, and interactions. As a result, he does not really know how the world works and what one is supposed to do in various situations. This can apply to even the smallest situations you might take for granted. Not knowing the unspoken rules of situations causes anxiety and upset. This leads to many of the behavioral issues that appear as the Asperger child tries to impose his own sense of order on a world he doesn't understand.

The Asperger child creates his own set of rules for everyday functioning to keep things from changing and thereby minimize his anxiety. Sometimes, he just makes up the rules when it is convenient. Other times, he attempts to make them up by looking for patterns, rules, or the logic of a situation to make it less chaotic for him and more predictable and understandable. If there are no rules for an event or situation, he will create them from his own experiences based on what he has read, seen, or heard. He will often have a great deal of information to use in reaching his conclusions and forming his opinions and feelings. As a result, some of his conclusions are correct and some are wrong.

He will rarely consider someone else's point of view if he does not consider them to be an "expert." The fewer people he sees as experts, the more behavioral difficulty you will see. He might consider teachers and others to be experts, but his parents will rarely be seen as such. Therefore, he will argue with you about your opinions if different from his own. He thinks that his opinion is as good as yours, so he chooses his. This represents his rigid thinking. He finds it difficult to be flexible and consider alternate views, especially if he has already reached a conclusion. New ideas can be difficult to accept ("I'd rather do it the way I've always done it"). Being forced to think differently can cause a lot of anxiety.

You must never overestimate your Asperger child's understanding of a situation because of his high intellectual ability or his other strengths. He is a boy who needs to figure out how the world works. He needs a road map and the set of instructions, one example at a time.

Frames of Reference

In trying to understand how the world works, your child tries to make sense of your explanations, but sometimes is not able to do this. As a result, your effort at intervening falls short. This can occur because your explanation has no meaning. Each Asperger child can only understand things for which they have a frame of reference, meaning they have a picture or idea about this from other sources or from prior discussions. They cannot understand what you will tell them without this frame of reference. For example, when I asked a teenaged boy if he missed his parents when he was at overnight camp for a week, he replied that it was not all that long. When I asked him again if he missed them, he said he could e-mail them whenever he wanted. After my third attempt to get an answer he finally said to me, "I can't answer that question. Since I have never missed anyone before, I have nothing against which I can compare my feelings to know what missing feels like." In the next few chapters we will explain how to give your child or teenager a new frame of reference.

Preferred and Nonpreferred Activities

For all Asperger individuals, life tends to be divided into two categories—preferred and nonpreferred activities. Preferred activities are those things he engages in frequently and with great intensity. He seeks them out without any external motivation. However, not all of his preferred activities are equal. Some are much more highly desired and prized. An activity that is lower on the list can never be used as a motivator for one that is higher. For example, you cannot get him to substitute his video game playing by offering a food reward if the game playing is higher on his list.

Any activity that is not preferred can be considered nonpreferred. They are less desirable and many are avoided. The lower they are on the list of desirability, the more he will resist or avoid doing them. Sometimes an activity or task becomes nonpreferred because it is made to compete with one that is much more highly valued. For example, taking a bath could be enjoyable, but if your child is reading, and reading is higher on his list, he will resist or throw a tantrum.

Preferred and nonpreferred activities are always problem areas. Your child or teen will always want to engage in preferred activities even when you have something more important for him to do. He does not want to end preferred activities and your attempts to have him end them can produce upset of one kind or another. On the other hand, trying to get him to do nonpreferred activities, such as interacting socially, can also be difficult. If many nonpreferred elements are combined together, the problem can become a nightmare, such as with homework.

The Asperger child rarely has activities he *just* likes. He tends to either love or hate an activity. The middle ground is usually missing. Teaching a middle ground or shades of gray can be a goal and will be discussed later. Also, as you try to teach him something new, you will encounter resistance because you are asking him to do something that's not a pre-ferred activity. But, as he outgrows younger interests, he will need to learn new ones in order to have some common interests with his peers. He needs to experience new things to see if he likes them, but may not want to do this just because you're asking him to do something new. He already has his list of preferred interests and will rarely see the need for anything new. Quite often, his preferred list will include computer or video games. However, the more he is on the computer or the more he plays video games, the less available he is to be in the real world and learn something new. Most likely, you will have to control his access to preferred activities if new ones are to be introduced.

Obsessive-Compulsive Behaviors and Anxiety

Obsessive-compulsive issues, also referred to as rituals, rigidity, perse-verations, rules, or black-and-white thinking, originate in the Asperger person's difficulty understanding the world around him. This creates anxiety, the underlying cause for his obsessive-compulsive behaviors. You will see anxiety in many different ways, depending on how your child manifests it. Some children will show it in obvious ways, such as crying, hiding under furniture, or clinging to you. Others show it by trying to control the situation and bossing people around. Some may hit or throw a tantrum. Some may act silly. No matter how your child displays his anxiety, you need to recognize that it is there and not as-sume it is due to some other cause such as attention seeking or just plain misbehavior.

Anxiety can occur for the smallest reason. Don't judge anxiety-producing situations by your own reaction to an event. Your child will be much more sensitive to situations than you will be, and often there will be no logical reason for his anxiety. Something that you would be anxious about causes no anxiety in your child, while a small event causes him to be quite anxious. When events change, he never knows what is going to come next and he becomes confused and upset, leading to some form of inappropriate behavior.

Your child's first reaction is to try to reduce or eliminate his anxiety. He must do something, and one of the most effective means is to take all changes, uncertainty, and variability out of the equation. This can be accomplished by obsessions. If everything is done a certain way, if there is a definite and unbreakable rule for every event, and if everyone does as he wishes, everything will be fine. Anxiety is then diminished or reduced, and no upset, tantrums, or meltdowns occur.

Unfortunately, it is virtually impossible to do this in the real world. Nevertheless, anxiety needs to be dealt with in some manner. This is the first order of business in planning for many interventions. If you move ahead before this has been settled, it will continue to be a significant interfering factor. Let's look at some examples of this.

Jack, age seventeen, won't leave the house because he wants to have his nails in a certain condition. This condition requires many hours of grooming that interfere with sleeping, eating, and doing just about anything else. This is obsessive-compulsive behavior. Any attempt to get him to leave the house or stop his nail maintenance causes anxiety and is rarely successful.

Anytime Mike, age eleven, hears an answer that he does not like, he becomes upset. If he asks a question or makes a request and the other person's response is not what he expected, he starts to argue with them, often acting out physically. He must have certain answers that are to his liking. This is rigidity in thought and it is also obsessive-compulsive.

Each of these cases has a cognitive and a behavioral component, and both must be considered. Each child must learn to get "unstuck" or let go of an issue and move on. They also need to learn how to change their thinking so that it doesn't become a problem to begin with. These details are provided in chapter 6. For more examples on how your child's anxiety may manifest itself, see the sidebar on page 35.

Black-and-White Thinking and Mindblindness

The obsessive-compulsive approach to life results in the narrow range of interests and insistence on set routines typical of an Asperger child. However, it usually starts as a cognitive (thinking) issue before it be-

BEHAVIORAL MANIFESTATIONS OF ANXIETY

• Reacting poorly to new events, transitions, or changes.

• Becoming easily overwhelmed and having difficulty calming down.

• Demonstrating unusual fears, anxiety, tantrums, and showing resistance to directions from others.

• Having a narrow range of interests, and becoming fixated on certain topics and/or routines.

• Insisting on having things and/or events occur in a certain way.

• Creating their own set of rules for doing something.

• Preferring to do the same things over and over.

• Wanting things to go their way, when they want them to, no matter what anyone else may want. They may argue, throw a tantrum, ignore you, growl, refuse to yield, etc.

• Having trouble playing and socializing well with peers or avoiding socializing altogether. They prefer to be alone because others do not do things exactly as they do.

• Lecturing others or engaging in a monologue rather than having a reciprocal conversation.

• Eating a narrow range of foods.

• Intensely disliking loud noises and crowds.

• Demanding unrealistic perfection in their handwriting, or wanting to avoid doing any writing.

• Tending to conserve energy and put forth the least effort they can, except with highly preferred activities.

• Remaining in a fantasy world a good deal of the time and appearing unaware of events around them.

• Displaying a good deal of silly behaviors because they are anxious or do not know what to do in a situation.

comes a behavioral one. Cognitive issues, such as the inability to take someone else's perspective (mindblindness) and the lack of cognitive flexibility (black-and-white thinking), cause many of the behaviors we see. We know there is a cognitive element by looking at the child's behaviors. There is always some distress, anxiety, or obsession manifested in every inappropriate behavior.

As mentioned, your child's cognitive difficulties lead to inaccurate interpretations and understanding of the world. How someone interprets a situation determines how he will respond to it. Many times the interpretation of an event is either not an accurate one or not one that leads to positive or prosocial actions. If the event can be reinterpreted for him, it might lead to a more productive outcome. In doing this, we must first try to understand how the individual interprets a situation. All of the individual's behaviors are filtered through his perception of the way the world works.

Take a look at the questions in the sidebar as they pertain to a problem situation. Try to answer all the questions to see which explanation fits the situation the best. Each of these questions represents a problematic way of thinking for your child. As a result of your questioning, it should become clearer that your child is engaging in a nonproductive interpretation and that correcting this faulty thinking with a more positive interpretation could lead to a more positive action. Remember, details are extremely important in trying to understand what is happening and what to do about it. Do not try to intervene until you understand, at least to a small degree, what is happening with your child. Changing thinking becomes a paramount issue, but one that is often neglected. However, successful changes in thinking will dramatically increase the success rate of any strategy you use.

Other Important Issues

Interest in Social Interactions

Basic social skills are usually very problematic. The Asperger child may look for the rules of social interactions, but they are never explicit.

QUESTIONS TO ASK ABOUT YOUR CHILD'S BEHAVIOR

To help you determine the reasons why your child acts the way he does, you should ask yourself the following questions:

1. Does he see only two choices to a situation rather than many options? (Black-and-white thinking.)

2. Because a situation was one way the first time, does he feel it has to be that way always? (Being rule bound.)

3. Is he misunderstanding what is happening and assuming something that isn't true? (Misinterpretation.)

4. Is he blaming you for something that is beyond your control? (He feels that you must solve the problem for him even when it involves issues you have no control over.)

5. Is he expecting perfection in himself? (Black-and-white thinking.)

6. Is he exaggerating the importance of an event? There are no small events, everything that goes wrong is a catastrophe. (Black-and-white thinking.)

7. Does he need to be taught a better way to deal with a problem? (He does not understand the way the world works.)

8. Has he made a rule that can't be followed? (He sees only one way to solve a problem. He cannot see alternatives.)

9. Is he stuck on an idea and can't let it go? (He does not know how to let go and move on when there is a problem.)

There are no specific rules about what to do, how to do it, when to do it, and so forth. He may look to categorize people to better understand them (e.g., "girls always talk a lot"). He will have difficulty taking others' perspectives or gauging others' feelings. However, we cannot overlook the degree of interest that your child has in being with peers. There are many Asperger children and adolescents who are indifferent to being with peers. They can take it or leave it. One moment they are enjoying the interaction and the next moment they have gone to their rooms to be alone, leaving a friend alone. Children who are less interested in others have less of a motivation to learn how to interact. Those who have a greater interest in others will be more willing to learn the social skills they need to relate to others. As a rule, your child will do better and have more interest in people he knows well; he will also do better with adults than with peers. Familiarity decreases his anxiety and may allow him to use skills he has already developed. If his anxiety is too great, he doesn't know what to say or how to say it.

Attention Deficit Hyperactivity Disorder (ADHD)

Most Asperger children have some degree of ADHD. This is not a separate disorder, but coexists with Asperger's syndrome. For some children this is a small issue marked by disorganization, forgetfulness, and lack of focus. For others, it can be a huge problem with issues that significantly affect his daily functioning. This is always an important issue and is often addressed through medication.

Sensory Issues Becoming Less Important

Sensory issues may have been a larger concern when your child was younger. Many Asperger children experience a reduction in their severity as they get older. A behavioral issue that may have initially been sensory may now be maintained due to habit or rigidity. Remember Noah and his issue of wearing clothes when in a car? Therefore, sensory concerns become less notable as explanations for behaviors, as well as targets for intervention.

Energy Conservation

Many Asperger children do not like to expend much energy. If they have a list of activities to choose from, they tend to select the ones that require the least amount of effort. For example, choosing between staying inside or going outside is often decided by which will be more tiring to do. Clearly, staying in will be selected. Reclining is often preferred to sitting up. Writing three lines is much better than a whole paragraph. Sports are avoided for multiple reasons. Conserving energy will often be a factor you encounter as you attempt to deal with certain issues.

Perfectionism

Many Asperger children are perfectionists in whatever they do. If they cannot be, they will not do the activity. Often they will look at something and can immediately tell if it will be too hard and the possibility for failure exists, and so they won't attempt it at all. This frequently occurs with homework, and is one of the reasons that homework is such an ordeal. This is one aspect of the black-and-white thinking we often see in the Asperger population. They see each mistake as a major error. Accidents, unintentional acts, misdemeanors, and bad judgment are all viewed as major felonies. It is very hard for them to see these situations as minor events. They need to learn, for instance, that some things are just an "oops," that they are not a very big deal and can easily be forgotten. This is part of their black-and-white thinking that was mentioned above. This issue must be addressed because life is filled with many situations that are quite trivial and should be treated as such.

Language

Your child may sound very adult with a large vocabulary. However, his language is too formal and it often sounds too old for his age. His voice quality is stilted and he lacks appropriate intonation. He is very literal and precise in his use of words and in noticing others' word usage. He can engage in a verbal exchange but gets stuck on certain feeling-related and abstract questions, and so does not answer them directly. Instead, he may say, "Enough of that." He will not say, "I don't know" very often. He will not often ask for help. The social aspects of language—using language for communication and interaction—are difficult. Higher order, abstract, feeling-related, and inferential questions are problematic. Basic language skills are excellent. Your interventions must always recognize the role of language.

Distress Issues

When your child gets overwhelmed, he does not tell anyone. He may try to avoid the problem altogether or may just growl. He may often be unaware of a problem if only others are affected by it, and so does nothing. Others may see his problems and may solve them for him. He tends to be rigid and "get stuck" with old, ineffective, and inefficient ways to solve a problem and cannot change his approach. He may fabricate stories about what happened when he is caught violating a rule. At such a time as this, he knows what the rule was, didn't follow it, and cannot find any other way out except by distorting the truth. Or he may not be able to give you a coherent explanation of what occurred. Those with Asperger's are rarely good reporters of events. The comings and goings of the day become confused and blend with events from another time or they may be presented out of sequence. In either case, he is upset about something, does not know how to effectively deal with the problem, has difficulty asking for help, and may act out in some way as a result. He will need to learn how to handle these stresses and distresses.

Internalizers and Externalizers

Some children with Asperger's *internalize* their problems. They become anxious or depressed. You are likely to hear comments from them such as, "I'm going to kill myself. I should never have been born. My life is worthless." When these comments occur, it is often because something upsetting has happened and they do not know how to deal with it. Most likely it is a very small problem that they have made into something monumental. They have "catastrophized" the problem. Rarely, if ever, do these children ever harm themselves. They threaten to do it, talk about it, but that is as far as it gets. Of course, it is scary for those who hear these comments, and it is very easy to overreact and consider them real threats. Nevertheless, always seek out professional advice in these situations, preferably from someone familiar with Asperger's.

Other children will become upset and threaten to harm others. They are going to kill someone, burn down the house or school, fire somebody, or do bodily harm. These are the *externalizers*. They will hit someone, throw an object, or do something similar, but they will rarely, if ever, cause murder—mayhem perhaps, but not murder. Yet again, it is difficult for those hearing these kinds of comments, and we recommend you seek professional help, again preferably from someone familiar with Asperger's.

School and Your Teenage Asperger Student

As your child becomes a preteen and teenager, socialization and behavioral issues continue to be the greatest needs. While they may be in mainstreamed settings in school, they are often misunderstood by their teachers and classmates, who attribute their behaviors to causes such as emotional disturbance or lack of motivation. It will be very important to help the school understand the needs of your child before issues occur. Be proactive in helping the staff learn how they can prevent problems. In all school settings, but especially those that are less structured, such as the cafeteria and the hallways, there is the potential for difficulty. The stress may build until there is a behavioral eruption of serious magnitude.

MIDDLE SCHOOL

In middle school, where there is the greatest pressure for conformity and the least tolerance for differences, Asperger students are frequently ignored, misunderstood, teased, or harassed. They may want to make friends and fit in more than ever, but are unable to because of their peculiarities and because they simply don't know how. These children may become withdrawn, act out, or be uncooperative, and are subject to various levels of depression. Other Asperger children can remain disinterested in fitting in, staying socially isolated, but still be the target of teasing and persecution by their peers. Coping skills are needed during this time more than at any other. A very important skill to learn will be "how to maintain a low profile" or not doing anything to draw attention to yourself. Making sure that your teen fits in and looks appropriate will help immensely.

Within the classroom, he may have learning deficits or may be on grade level. You may need to ask for special accommodations within the classroom to allow some degree of success for your Asperger student. These may be academic, behavioral, or organizational. Some assignments will be very difficult to do because of neurological deficits. Your teenager may not be able to volunteer in class or make a presentation in front of the class. Keeping track of assignments, turning in homework, and doing long-term projects may all prove overwhelming unless addressed through accommodations and skill development prior to and during this time period. If your child is a good student, he will often show a lot of interest in some area and excel in it. These areas are often mathematics, computers, and related subjects. At the same time, he may have difficulty with certain aspects of the curriculum. This includes misunderstanding material, especially when it involves abstractions, idioms, opinions, feelings, and/or preferences. Inattention and organizational difficulties may exist for those who are otherwise academically able as well as those who are less so.

The "hidden curriculum" of the school tends to elude Asperger students. These teenagers have a hard time following the school rules, let alone the more subtle issues of how the school community operates. Helping him to know this "hidden curriculum" is another important goal for you to work on.

HIGH SCHOOL

By high school age, your Asperger teen's peculiarities might be better tolerated by his peers. However, there may still be other kids who will tease your teen. If your teen displays significant academic talent in some area, there is a chance for some peer respect. More likely, he may find other students who share similar interests, such as computers, science, or some other preferred activities. There is always a group of students who are seen as "nerds" or "geeks" who will accept the Asperger student if he has similar interests. Try to find this group in your school. It is very important that your Asperger teenager develop coping skills, social skills, and the ability to fit into some subgroup of the general high school population. If he is not able to do this, his risk for depression increases. To this end, a mentor, whether it is a peer or an adult, is necessary to help your student learn the skills that are necessary for survival in high school. This will be a critical part of this student's curriculum.

There is also another group of Asperger students who continue to experience difficulties, become unable to manage their anxiety, and drop out of school. For them, school becomes an intolerable place that is to be avoided at all costs. These people may also have too much anxiety to seek and hold a job. For them, it becomes imperative that you recognize their anxiety and turmoil and help them manage it before it reaches this crisis stage.

At home, you will have all the teenage issues along with Asperger issues. Don't try to distinguish which is which. Any inappropriate behavior is important to deal with. Unfortunately, the teenager with Asperger's is the hardest age group to deal with. Emotional reactions become more significant and additional skills will need to be taught. Your teenager may not know how to have a discussion, how to compromise or negotiate. These are skills you will need to teach him before he becomes a teenager.

As the years unfold, the likelihood for medication increases in order to manage some of the symptoms associated with Asperger's. These include anxiety, obsessive-compulsive behaviors, depression, and aggression. Working with a good psychiatrist often becomes a crucial component to getting through the teen years.

Determining Triggers for the Behavior

Once you have reasons for the behavior, you are ready for the next step—determining what triggers your child's general behavior. You need to determine what issues occur most frequently. For example, is there usually a problem at dinner, when doing homework, or about shutting off the computer? Do disappointments and surprises create problems for your child? Which new situations or changes cause anxiety? Is there a problem going to restaurants or stores? These events will become the targets for your intervention.

As an example, whenever Ruth, age six, went into a store with her mother, she would begin to whine and complain about wanting to leave after a few minutes. She would do this even if she wasn't tired or hungry. The behavior always began a few minutes after entering a store, although it rarely occurred in a store that Ruth wanted to be in. No matter how many times her mother told her she had to wait, it continued. Now, this may seem like typical behavior for a six-year-old, and you may be right. However, what makes an Asperger child different is that, this behavior is more intense, more frequent, and lasts longer than it would in a typical six-year-old. Ruth's behavior seemed to be the result of three issues: wanting to end a nonpreferred activity, not knowing how to do it appropriately, and what to do when she still had to participate in a nonpreferred activity.

Roger, age seven, would touch things that belonged to other people wherever he was. This included while waiting to check his book out at the library, when he was finished with his work in class, or when he was finished playing in my office and was getting ready to leave. Roger did not know what to do when he had to structure his time and actions, and he needed to learn this skill.

As you can see, once you have generated a hypothesis for the behavior, what needs to be done becomes clearer. Ruth needed to understand the rules of being in a store, how to wait, and how to know when it is time to leave. Roger needed to know what to do when he has free time or is waiting for the next activity. In both cases, they had to learn replacement skills, which will be discussed in chapters 5 and 6.

This chapter has discussed many of the issues that determine the behaviors you see, as well as the thinking that your child or teen experiences that makes him different from the typical child or teen. As you read on, it will be very helpful to remember these points as you try to understand how your child sees the world. Consider which of these characteristics your child has. As you realize how he sees the world, you will be able to predict how he will act. Increasing your understanding of his world will enable you to really help him.

3

Identifying Asperger Subtypes

"They're Not All the Same."

Ten-year-old Kenny cried and hid under furniture at the drop of a hat. On picture day at school, when there was something new for dinner, because Mom was not waiting at the bus stop—all were reasons for considerable upset. When he came to see me at my office, for many weeks he cried, yelled, and hid. After a period of time, Kenny got used to seeing me, but other new things continued to upset him.

We devised a plan. The next time he came to see me I would take him into the community and he would experience something new, and we would continue this each week. At first, he was quite opposed to doing it. We wrote out an agreement about what and how we would do this. It became very clear to him what was expected, where we would go, and every other detail. Finally, he agreed. He was so certain he would do it that he told me to just show him the card on which we had written all the details and he would be fine.

On the day of our first journey, his mother came into my office, shaking her head. All was not right. Kenny came in behind her looking quite forlorn. I soon learned he had not slept for three nights, dreading our forthcoming trip. Telling his mother not to worry, I took him into my office and confidently showed him the card we had created the week before. He took one look at the card and ripped it to shreds.

After his considerable crying and yelling, we were able to talk about good choices and bad choices. We talked about conquering our fears. Nothing helped. Then it finally dawned on me: Kenny didn't respond to rules about what he was supposed to do. He didn't care if he was prepared for the outing. He didn't even care when I explained my reasons for doing this. He was not a "Logic Boy" or a "Rule Boy." He was an "Anxiety Boy." Reasons didn't matter. I had to come up with a new plan that recognized his emotions would always get in the way of his thinking. Through trial and error, I came up with the idea of beginning his office visit differently. We met outside my office rather than in it, so that he wouldn't have to leave my office to go to somewhere. This seemed better to him and made him feel less anxious, and we made our first trip to Starbucks for a soda and a doughnut, both of which he loved.

Changing the sequence of events can sometimes change the outcome. After our first success, others were easier even though anxiety was still present. I used forced choices, so that he had to do things despite some anxiety. I could not let him avoid learning to deal with new situations. Sometimes you cannot reduce anxiety to zero before you attempt something new or different.

The new plan finally worked well and we went on to many other new adventures in Dr. Sohn's neighborhood.

Asperger "Subtypes"

It is important to recognize that each Asperger child is different, with his or her own unique set of issues. No two are exactly the same. However, there are three main subtypes: the Rule Boy, the Logic Boy, and the Emotion Boy, each with its own basic set of issues and several individual subtypes. It is very important to clarify each child's issues, because each type demands a different kind of response from you. Choosing the right approach is crucial if changes are to occur. By determining your child's type you will be able to identify his most important characteristics and learn what his core issues are. This helps to determine where to begin the treatment program. Once the type is identified, the basic issues for each will become clear and the course of action can be specified. The course of action consists of teaching the various skills that are lacking or replacing those skills that are inappropriate.

Although Asperger children differ from others by their worldview and many other ways we've already discussed, the primary issue to be determined is his individual *coping strategy*. Each child has developed a very specific way to deal with problem situations, and his particular strategy determines the subtype to which he belongs.

The Rule Boy

Having a set of rules to live by is the most important issue for this type. Once he has a set of rules to follow, there tend to be few, if any, concerns, except in areas where you have not yet established rules. If there is a void where a rule has not been established, the Rule Boy is not happy; because he doesn't know what to do in that situation, he makes up his own rules. Any situation that has too few rules will be a bad one for this type of child. He must have rules to live by and he will create his own if you don't provide them, which will probably not match what others are thinking. This will cause conflict and upset until someone prevails and the rules are clarified. This boy respects authority figures and does well when it is perfectly clear who is in charge and who makes the rules. This child can often be fine in school but a real problem at home, because the rules are not clear enough in the latter situation. It is not unusual for parents of this type to be quite surprised to hear how well behaved their child is in school. There are two main subtypes of Rule Boy—the innocent/passive and the overcontrolled—but not every one has all of the characteristics listed below.

INNOCENT/PASSIVE BOY

This child or teen is often seen as a teacher's delight. Everywhere he goes, others remark how well behaved he is. He is never a discipline problem, never a disruption. However, at home his behaviors can be terrible. He can be quite bossy and controlling. Tantrums, yelling, and arguing can be a daily occurrence. The key to recognizing this type is the behavior differences between home and school. If he is poorly behaved in school as well, he is not a Rule Boy.

The Rule Boy wants to please others. He doesn't want anyone mad at him. He is very cooperative with authority figures and is very obedient, often to a fault. He can be too naive and taken advantage of because he will be reluctant to stand up for himself or be assertive. He tries to "fly under the radar." He does not want to stand out. While his behavior is unusually good, he can become distressed by others who do not follow the rules. Often, these children monitor others' actions and will "tell on them," becoming the "rule police." Clearly, these children have anxiety, but it is not overwhelming for them. They manage their anxiety by following the rules and making sure others do as well. Problems only occur for them when rules are absent or vague and the person in charge lacks authority in their eyes.

Recommended Approach: Structure, routines, schedules, and prompting cards are some of the tools used to create a new set of appropriate rules for this child in every difficult setting no matter how small the situation might be. There is no such thing as a situation that is too small to have rules. Going to a store, taking a bath, deciding where to eat dinner— all need rules. You need to supply a set of rules regarding appropriate behaviors to be demonstrated in each problem situation, and state them like this: "The rule is . . ." Don't hesitate to also explain why you are doing what you are doing. This will help generalize these skills later on.

For example, you would say, "The rule is, when we take a bath we can only put ten toys in the tub" (or whatever number you think is right). "We'll stay in the tub for twenty minutes, and when the buzzer goes off it's time to get out and we'll go in your room and put your pj's on. We'll go back in the bathroom and brush your teeth for two minutes and then get back in bed and we'll read one book before we shut the lights out and go to bed." These rules can be modified to suit your particular situation, but it should give you an idea of the details that may be needed for your child.

Highly structured classrooms run by authority figures won't need to do much of this. Instead, they will be trying to help the rule child be less rule bound and have greater tolerance for ambiguity.

OVERCONTROLLED BOY

This is another type of Rule Boy, who is very similar to the above sub-type, except his behavior is good at home as well as at school. He is also rule bound, with rules for everything. He has learned to control outbursts, sometimes too much, in all situations. In this case, he sees his parents, who have created many rules for him to follow at home, as authority figures just like his teachers. There are no situations that don't have rules for him to follow. All other characteristics from above are similar, and he, too, is far and away overly obedient. He needs to become more flexible.

Recommended Approach: You won't have to worry about rules with this girl or boy. You need to begin a crash course in flexibility to help him see the world as less black-and-white. He will need to learn much more about the reasons behind actions and how the world works, with less emphasis on obedience. Don't throw out the rules altogether, but slowly help him to learn decision-making and problem-solving skills so he can become a more independent thinker.

The Logic Boy

This child or teen needs to know the reasons for the rules before he is okay. Blindly accepting your rules is not the way he operates. He wants to know the reasons behind your actions, why something is done a certain way, and it has to make sense to him. If it seems too arbitrary, it's not an adequate reason in his mind, and he won't listen. His coping strategy is to try to make sense of the world through logic, reasoning, and rational thought. He wants the world to be a place with order and rationality to it. This reduces his anxiety. He may ask lots of questions about how the world works. He uses his very well-developed logical mind to understand what is going on, and you need to give him the reasoning behind a decision or an action.

He is often a very bright boy with a high IQ. He usually becomes more flexible when he knows the reason for something. The rule alone is not sufficient. After you have explained the reason for your request, many behavioral issues decrease. However, he may not accept your logic unless it is quite convincing, because he may very well have his own reasons and explanations. His view of the world is based on logic and reasons, which can also cause him to become overanalytical. In this case, he often cannot function appropriately because he never gets past the analysis stage to the action stage. He suffers from "analysis paralysis." Remember, not every Logic Boy has all of these characteristics.

Recommended Approach: You will need to explain why something needs to be done or why it can't be done before you will get compliance. For the Logic Boy, understanding precedes cooperation. If your explanations provide him with information he didn't have, might have overlooked, or didn't understand, you will have helped him clarify the way the world works and how a desired action is beneficial to him. As these children become older, you will need to do much more explaining because rules by themselves will have less impact. As you explain things to these children, always match your explanation to their cognitive and emotional level. Don't overestimate how much they know because they have a large vocabulary. Always make sure they understand you as you move step by step. As you explain something from a new angle you will help them see it differently. For those who overanalyze, you will have to help them reduce the amount of analysis by helping them see how it is unproductive. Let's look at an example:

Matt was an eight-year-old who always came home from school hungry. Each day he walked in the front door and began to argue with his mother about dinner. He wanted it right away and couldn't wait for her to finish it. These battles led to knock-down, drag-out fights, culminating in Mom pinning Matt to the floor. After going through this struggle on a daily basis, Mom sought help. As always, we discussed the particulars, gathered information, listened to all sides of the problem, and then began our discussion. It went something like this:

DR. S.: So, Matt, it seems you come into the house pretty hungry, don't you?

MATT: Yes, I do.

DR. S.: And after arguing with Mom, it becomes a real fight, with you guys rolling around on the floor. Kicking and screaming.

MATT: That sounds like it.

DR. S.: When Mom is down on the floor with you, she's of course still stirring and mixing and working on preparing dinner, isn't she?

MATT: (*A long pause*) Oh, I get it. Of course not. She's on the floor with me.

DR. S.: You mean that wrestling with her doesn't get your dinner finished any quicker?

MATT: How can it?

DR. S.: Well, that's the point, Matt. It can't, can it? It probably causes a real delay in getting dinner ready instead. Just what you didn't want.

MATT: I guess it doesn't help.

DR. S.: You guess it doesn't help? Let me spell it out for you. Choice one: You come in the house and calmly and quickly work out a solution with Mom about your hunger and she can finish getting dinner ready. Choice two: You come in and fight with her. Dinner is not done quickly, but instead takes even longer to get ready. You wind up upset, without food, and having to wait even longer for it to be ready. Hmmm. Sounds like a really tough choice to make.

MATT: I get this, but what am I supposed to do when I come home and I'm really hungry?

DR. S.: How about if the three of us come up with a list of foods you could eat then that won't ruin your appetite and will allow mom to finish dinner?

MATT: Okay.

DR. S.: Let's write up this list and call it "a little something." That way, when you come home and you're hungry, Mom can say, "Matt, why don't you take 'a little something' to eat?" and you'll both know what this means without arguing.

MATT: This sounds like a good idea.

We then drew up a written list on a three-by-five-inch index card, which he took home (and which we reviewed the next week to see if it worked—it did). And the fighting ended.

The Emotion Boy

This is the most difficult type to deal with because rules and reasons mean much less to him or her. Many of the Asperger children fall into one of the emotion types. Their emotions control their behaviors. If you do not recognize and deal with their emotions, your success is diminished. This group has many more tantrums, is less available, easily disengages, or is more prone to acting out. Those dealing with the Emotion Boy can often find themselves in a state of frustration at best and a crisis state at worst. The vast majority of this group will end up on medications for their issues because their coping strategies are poorly developed and inadequate to meet the demands of the world. Fortunately, the right medication and an effective behavioral plan can do wonders.

PARANOID BOY

By far, this is the most difficult type. Fortunately, their numbers are small. Some other subtypes may have characteristics similar to this type, but not all. He sees the world from an adversarial point of view. The world is against him. Everyone is out to get him and no one can be trusted. The only coping strategy he has is to maintain a good "offense" and so he attacks before others do or say anything. Even the slightest issue is a source of provocation. Once he begins his attack he can be relentless, and keep coming at you until he is exhausted. If he is younger, you might have the stamina to deal with this. If he is older, the police are often called. These children are unusually bright. Their thinking involves violent themes and their actions are hostile and aggressive to others. They want to "fire, murder, devour, shoot, destroy" people who go against them in any situation, no matter how trivial. Typically, they receive multiple diagnoses, often oppositional defiant disorder or some other psychiatric condition such as bipolar disorder.

Recommended Approach: Since this is the most difficult type by far, you must take extraordinary means to help these children. Placating your child or "walking on eggshells" will only give you a momentary reprieve. Most parents of these children refrain from physical interventions, but may be using a good deal of restraining techniques. This again is a temporary solution. To begin with, you must seek professional help, in terms of both medication and behavioral interventions. You must maintain calmness in your interactions with these children. Only the most powerful reinforcers may be of some use. A highly structured environment with firmness is needed, along with great persistence and patience. Dealing with this type is something you don't do alone.

ADHD, OCD, AND FANTASY CHILDREN

The factors marking these three subtypes—attention deficit hyperactivity disorder (ADHD), obsessive-compulsive disorder (OCD), and preoccupation with a fantasy world—are very closely related, even intertwined. In all three, the child is often described as being inattentive, but there are a number of reasons for the inattention. If he is an ADHD child, he is inattentive because he is *nowhere*. He is not focused on any one thing for very long. He is distracted by anything new or different that passes in front of his eyes, and his interest moves from one thing to another and he cannot easily control his focus. He has many of the other signs of ADHD as well. He is easily distracted, disorganized, forgetful, and impulsive. He may or may not be hyperactive.

The OCD child, on the other hand, is inattentive because he is *somewhere else*. He is not so much distracted as preoccupied with something else that is of greater interest to him, usually related to some preferred activity such as videos, numbers, or how things are placed in his environment. Some children have one or the other, ADHD or OCD, and most have both to varying degrees. Since symptoms of both disorders can exist at the same time and to varying degrees, it can be difficult to tell which is which at times. In either case, the result is a lack of awareness of what is going on around him. However, it is important to distinguish between the two and decide how much each contributes to the inattention, because your approach for each will be different. Underfocusing (predominantly

ADHD) and overfocusing (predominantly OCD) are important variables that must be addressed, as well as the child who dwells in a fantasy world.

PREDOMINATELY ADHD

This child is very unfocused and has difficulty attending to and processing information on a consistent basis. He is easily distracted and forgetful, loses things, and has significant difficulty keeping track of school assignments. He wanders around in the classroom and may not be able to stay in his seat at home and in school. Conversations are difficult because he is always looking around the room at something else, but doesn't stay focused on any one thing very long.

Recommended Approach: Medication is very important to deal with inattention and impulsiveness. Careful monitoring of all tasks and situations, along with powerful reinforcers, is sometimes helpful. He will find it hard to stay focused on most tasks. Frequent breaks, structured tasks, and supervision are all necessary. If you find the right medication, the inattention reduces significantly, but may not disappear.

PREDOMINATELY OCD

This child has many obsessions that take him elsewhere, away from the here and now. Although he appears inattentive, in reality, he has other issues that he is dealing with instead. For example, are his shoelaces tied the way he likes them? Is everything around him exactly where it belongs? How many dots are in that ceiling tile over his head? Did he ask the question that he wanted to in the right way? And so on. The list can be endless. But no matter what is on his list, it usually takes precedence over anything that is on your list. He is often a perfectionist, and everything has to go a certain way. If it doesn't, it's the end of the world. There is no middle ground; everything is black or white. It is either perfect or it is terrible.

He may have completion rituals where things must be finished before he moves on. And there are many rituals or routines in this child's life. For example, he can't shut off his Game Boy until he reaches a certain level or he can't shut off the TV until the program is totally and completely over. All of this and more can be going on in his head and cause him to disengage from reality and become unavailable.

Let's look at an example: Tommy, age seven, only wants to play his video games. He always plays them after dinner until bedtime. When he is playing them, he finds it very hard to stop. He argues, whines, and may even have a tantrum when asked to try an alternative to video game playing. He has certain requirements for getting ready for bed and an order to them. He changes his clothes under his covers, even though there is no one else in his room. He brushes his teeth for 120 seconds. Mom has to kiss him good night first, Dad is next, and then he gets a story that he always picks from the books on his shelf. He has to have his radio on in order to fall asleep because he has to hear the music and have the light from the radio shining in his room. Tommy has lots of rules about how things are supposed to go in his world. He is an OCD child. Now, it may seem like he is a Rule child with all of these rules, but there is a difference. The Rule child will typically follow others' rules once they are spelled out to him. The OCD child makes up his own rules about everything and only wants to follow his own rules, no one else's. The OCD child is compelled by his anxiety to follow his own dictates: he must be in control. The Rule child's anxiety compels him to follow everyone else's: he must obey. Each has a different motivation and therefore a different response.

Recommended Approach: You must gain control over his obsessions. There must be limits and restrictions on certain activities. Rituals and routines are addressed through sabotage, which will be discussed in chapter 6. You must teach him how to be more flexible by changing routines. You must expand his repertoire of interests, teach him shades of gray, and have him develop a balance in his life. Obsessions will remain, but you can use them as reinforcers as long as you limit the amount of time spent on the obsessions. Each of these things is discussed later on.

PREDOMINATELY FANTASY
This child is very similar to the OCD type except his distractions primarily involve his preoccupations with fantasy. This means Game Boy,

Nintendo, Xbox, video games, Pokémon, Yu-Gi-Oh!, the Cartoon Network, TV shows, Japanese animé, fantasy books, show tunes—the list is endless, but often involves electronics in some way. Not only does he obsess over the use of the electronic equipment, but the fantasy reoccurs without it as well. If the fantasy involves books or music, he doesn't need the actual object to experience its pleasure. So he replays, recreates, or in some way engages in the obsession in his head. As he is eating dinner, sitting in class, doing his homework, or talking to you, there is another tape playing in his head. And this tape is all about fantasy. He does word-for-word scripting of dialogue and scenes in his head, combines different ones together, or makes up his own based on something he has seen or read. He may have many other obsessions, but the strongest are about fantasies. These fantasies serve many functions—besides being very enjoyable, they remove him from the unpleasantness of the real world, demands are reduced, and everything goes just the way he wants. As a result, reality is avoided, interactions with others don't occur, and life goes on without him. This is how he copes with stress and reality. Interfere with his preoccupations and you will experience his wrath. Leave him to his preoccupations and he can amuse himself for hours.

Recommended Approach: Everything we said about the OCD type applies here. Additionally, you must go beyond those techniques to include teaching him the difference between reality and fantasy—how to recognize it, what constitutes each, and how to be in the here and now. You must limit fantasy time and help him to develop the ability to enjoy nonfantasy activities (this is one of the many goals of the techniques discussed in the coming chapters). If he can't enjoy the real world, he won't want to be a part of it. Medication is almost always necessary.

ANXIETY BOY
This child differs from all other types because he has no coping strategy. While every other type experiences anxiety to some degree, they cope with it through rules, rituals, obsessions, or fantasy. The Anxiety

Boy has never figured out how to deal with problems. As a result, his anxiety overwhelms him and he shuts down, hides under furniture, cries, wants to stay at home, acts silly, wants to stay inside, and tries to avoid people and places outside of his small comfort zone. In other words, he becomes a mess. He is very rigid but doesn't really know the rules of the world. His anxiety comes from his confusion and lack of understanding of how the world works. He just doesn't get it.

He usually needs much more time to handle even the smallest issue. You cannot give him too many issues to deal with at once, even if they are all small, or he will be overwhelmed. Bigger issues are too much as well and he falls apart. Sometimes the issues are so small that you think they cannot possibly cause a problem. Not true. Even the smallest change can result in upset if his anxiety is too big. The degree of anxiety varies, and not all children have the same amount, and not all situations produce the same degree of upset. He can be upset if it's picture day at school, his teacher is absent, someone comes to visit his parents at home, he has to get his hair cut, you give him the orange cheese and not the yellow cheese—this list can be longer than any other list we've talked about because everything has the potential to be upsetting. You'll know you have an Anxiety Boy because he cries quite a bit, clings to you in new situations or with new people, doesn't want to leave his house, and when away from home often tells you he wants to go back home immediately. His tantrums end when he is allowed to be alone in his room under the covers. Once he gets used to something he can often do better. So once he is desensitized to school, he can be okay if he sees it as a structured, calm, and safe place. He, too, may then act better at school than at home, or he may be the same in both places.

Recommended Approach: This boy or girl needs a great deal of structure, routine, and explanation about every possible troublesome situation. You need to explain the rules of each situation, including what to do and what not to do, before he experiences the situation. You need to give him lots of warning on what is going to happen, preparing him for change. Never overwhelm him. Go slowly and don't try to accomplish too much at one time. Help him get past each issue that has occurred, to get "over it" and move on, or they will build up and the next small one will cause him to fall apart. These are the prevention aspects of dealing with anxiety. That is, you will try to prevent situations from overwhelming him. However, that will never be sufficient and he will need to learn how to cope with it as well. Teach stress management skills: stress resiliency, stress immunity, learned optimism, and "theory of mind." Teach him emotional regulation skills: anxiety management, self-calming, being okay, and the like. (See pages 118–135.) Medication may be needed if these skills are difficult for him to learn.

ANGRY/RESISTANT BOY

This child or teen may look similar to the paranoid type, but he is less adversarial and less intense. He is also easier to deal with if and when he feels safer. He argues about everything, and almost anything can lead to a tantrum of some size. At times, he can be violent and physical or will destroy property. He wants things to go his way. He wants to control situations and has his own rules about the world and how things are supposed to be. He is often diagnosed with oppositional defiant disorder (ODD). This is another child who doesn't understand the way the world works and becomes anxious as a result. He feels threatened by others and thinks they are trying to control him or are being unfair and arbitrary. He needs to fight with them to gain control and get things straightened out to his way of thinking. However, his arguing does nothing but further aggravate the situation. His rigidity, lack of understanding, and disuse of logic prevent him from seeing this clearly. His emotions determine his actions.

Recommended Approach: Try to avoid power struggles. Do not show much emotion in your responses and try to be matter-of-fact. Stay focused on a particular issue and don't get sidetracked as you have a discussion with this child. It's very easy for the discussion to get off track and become nonproductive. Try to see his arguing as a sign of anxiety and not purposeful misbehavior. Try to get him to see you as a helper or problem solver rather than an adversary or problem causer. Don't overfocus on the content of a discussion, but rather on the process; that is, what is going on behind the content of the discussion.

For example, a discussion may begin around what he is going to get from you for Christmas. Before you know it, you are being accused of buying others bigger and better presents. Or perhaps the accusation is that you never buy him what he really wants. Rather than debate the merits of this argument, which will only escalate further, you should discuss how he is stuck on certain ideas that will only lead to greater upset, and the impact his actions have on himself and others. He must begin to see his role in what is going on and stop blaming others for what occurs. You will need to teach him how to stay focused and how to self-calm, as well as how to compromise and negotiate. But most of all, he needs to see you as trying to help him solve his problems, not making them worse. (See chapters 5 and 8.)

NEGATIVE BOY

This child or teen tends to be more of an annoyance than anything else. He does a lot of complaining and whining about doing things that are not preferred activities because he only enjoys preferred activities. As a result of his actions, there can be a good deal of arguing and refusals. He usually sees the world in a negative way—"the glass is half empty"—and rarely sees the good aspects of an event or situation, no matter how much good has occurred. Tantrums, bossiness, rituals, and rules are not issues. He may even be fairly cooperative at times. The major concern regarding this child is that he is more prone to future depression than any other type.

Recommended Approach: He must learn to be okay with nonpreferred activities and that it is better to "say nothing than be negative." You need to teach her how to use positive commenting and responses. Direct instruction in how to have a "positive attitude" and "learned optimism" (see pages 121–122) is needed.

Each child can have many issues that make him unique. In this chapter and the last, you have begun to sort out those factors that make your child who he is. It is his uniqueness that tells you what subtype he is and what techniques you need to use. When you understand your child and his interaction with the world, you will be better able to help him reach his full potential. If you still are not sure of the subtype characteristics your child demonstrates, at least provide the two things every Asperger child needs: structure and predictability. These are discussed in the next chapter.

4

Structure and Predictability

THE FOUNDATION FOR CHANGE

"I'm Flexible, I Just Don't Like Change"

Over the years, we have discovered there are many food issues for Asperger children. If one child vomits during lunch, there will be at least one other with a sensitive gag reflex who will immediately vomit in response. Always being preventive and, in this case, out of true necessity (the less vomit to clean up, the better), I needed to develop a "vomit rule." The vomit rule was: As soon as someone vomits, you look away and think about your favorite thing. Do not turn back around until you are told to do so. Since almost all children with Asperger's syndrome have a favorite obsession that they are usually told not to think about, adding this detail made this strategy especially appealing. With this strategy in place, I felt confident. However, whenever a new group of children come together this rule needs to be reintroduced. The first day of school in my first-grade class is a very busy one for the children. Unfortunately, with so many rules to learn, the vomit rule was overlooked on our first visit to the cafeteria. When you fail to prevent a particular response, that is usually when it will occur.

One of the children was eating yogurt and, without warning, vomited. My old students, on cue, immediately turned their heads and looked out the window. As I turned to help the child who vomited, the child next to him threw up. Now on alert, I see another child beginning to gag. I turn and say the following, in my rules voice, "The rule is, only two children can vomit at the same time." The third child did not vomit. In the Asperger world, a rule is a rule.

Prevention strategies are used not just to avoid tantrums and meltdowns, but to prevent situations from getting out of hand. Though I had not taught the vomit rule, I had taught that school was a place with rules and when the teacher says, "This is a rule; we have to follow it." Prevention: it's how you play the game.

Creating Stable Conditions for Learning

A primary goal of Cognitive Social Integration Therapy is to stabilize events and emotions to create an atmosphere that will allow progress. Tantrums, upset, resistance, and arguments need to be reduced to an acceptable level. To accomplish this goal you must begin to prevent problems that may occur during the normal part of everyday life, such as getting ready for school, eating meals, going on family excursions, doing homework, getting ready for bed, playing with peers, following school rules, and so on. Situations of this kind must be dealt with before you can do anything else. If this goes badly, you will not be able to tackle more difficult situations.

In this chapter you will learn how to reduce problems and increase compliance by thinking about problems in a different way. Instead of reacting after an event, you will begin to think about situations before they occur and become more proactive in trying to prevent a problem situation. You will also realize you have a role in what happens with your child, not necessarily in causing a problem, but in increasing or decreasing it. Finally, you will see that details are very important in understanding, planning, and executing any interventions.

To create a calmer overall atmosphere that will serve as a platform for further future gains, you should embrace a number of useful practices:

1. Analyzing your child's behavior

2. Selecting and prioritizing goals

3. Preventing problems rather than reacting to them

4. Using environmental controls, including consistency and reinforcers

5. Using language, including key words and phrases

6. Using visuals, including schedules

7. Special considerations for the teenage years

Analyzing Your Child's Behavior

Effective interventions are based on a step-by-step approach. As a result, you will need to know where to begin. After you have collected data (such as through the evaluation aids in appendices A and B) and identified the areas of difficulty, you must identify specific examples and situations where a given difficulty manifests itself. Select a very clear and simple situation, such as interrupting or not coming to dinner. Gather all the details about that example—what happens before, during, and after the event. Think about what went wrong and how it should go correctly—in other words, what skills are lacking in your child. Assume that she does not know the correct behavior and/or does not understand why that behavior needs to occur. What does your child need to know to do this activity or task in a better way? Help her to understand the rules for the situation and the reasons for the rules. The latter puts the rules into a context and helps with generalization later on. Many times people just tell a child what not to do, but leave out what she is supposed to do. Figuring out what to do is not easy; that is what you will learn how to impart to her in this chapter.

Selecting and Prioritizing Goals

In selecting a target goal (see the Levels of Interventions diagram on page 66), it is better to choose something that is small and has a high frequency of occurrence. In this way, you can repeatedly practice on the same event until it has been mastered. Do not choose the goal that is the most important or the biggest. These will meet with the most resistance

LEVELS OF INTERVENTIONS

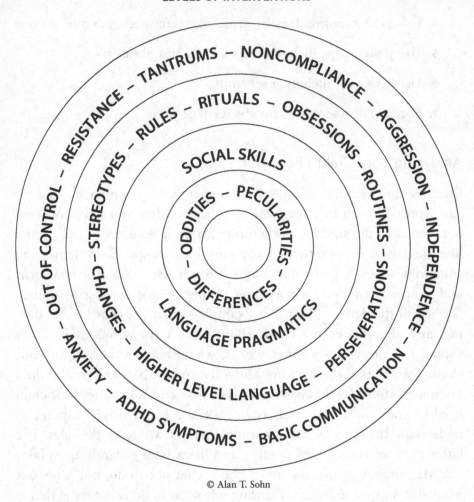

© Alan T. Sohn

from your child, and addressing smaller goals first will eventually lead to larger ones. Also, it is important to recognize that you must be consistent and address the targeted goal each time it occurs. Change it step by step and deal with every detail of it. This is a process as much as it is an end result. How it is done is of more value, at first, than your outcome. Learn from it as you are doing it. Issues on the outer ring of the Levels of

Interventions diagram need to be addressed and mastered before those in the inner circles.

Preventing Problems Rather Than Reacting to Them

Sooner is better than later. Most people tend to wait until a problem arises and then attempt to deal with it through the use of a consequence. Consequences can be positive (gaining something) or negative (losing something). At times, consequences are discussed prior to an event, but usually in terms of a motivator: "If you do this, you will gain [lose] something else." More often we use consequences in the middle of a problem, such as, "If you don't stop that, you're going right to bed." Or, "You won't watch any TV if you don't leave your sister alone." Or, "You're in time-out right now. I've had it." All of these statements are made when the behavior is out of control. You have given many warnings and you are now acting out of frustration. However, none of these comments will lead to positive change in the short or long run.

With an Asperger child it is far better to anticipate the occurrence of a behavior and then plan for it. Many problem behaviors are repetitious, especially in the same situation. Even when they don't occur every time, they may still be frequent enough to warrant this approach. A rule of thumb is if a behavior repeats itself at least half of the time, you need to prepare for it. For example, if homework, bedtime, or dinnertime have been frequent problems in the past, chances are very good they will continue to be so in the future.

Future vision is the ability of an individual to know what is going to happen in an upcoming situation because of its constant reoccurrence. When you know what is going to happen you can prepare your child for the event prior to its occurrence by discussing what usually occurs and what needs to occur. For example, going out to dinner is often a problem time. So talk with your child about what normally happens, how he acts, how you do, and then follow that up with a discussion and see if you can get a firm commitment from your child that he is going to follow these new behaviors. If he responds in a positive way, you have increased the likelihood that things will go better when you go out for dinner.

If you happen to miss the opportunity to prevent a problem, there is often a small "window of opportunity" in which you can still salvage the situation. In the example above, suppose you have forgotten to say something before you left for dinner. As events begin to unravel, you have a very brief period of time—sometimes only a minute or two—before you'll be in a messy situation. Seize this opportunity. It may be the last best one in that situation.

Using Environmental Controls

To make interventions effective you need to create an environment in which your child feels comfortable, anxiety is decreased, and your child has an understanding of the events taking place around him. The environment needs to provide consistency, predictability, structure, routine, organization, logically explained rules, and clear rewards/consequences in response to these rules. When this is in place, your child will begin to feel competent. I am reminded of a student who had been expelled from his kindergarten class as the result of unmanageable behaviors—even with one-on-one support. After his first week in my class of eight Asperger students, without any additional support, he said, "Hey, I like this new school. I know the way." A number of things must be in place to create "the Asperger world."

PHYSICAL ENVIRONMENT
First, the physical environment must be consistent. In all locations you need to identify consistent areas where specific activities are completed, such as that homework is always completed at the desk in his bedroom or at the kitchen table. These areas/activities should also have consistent behavioral expectations, which are explained to your child, such as, "At my desk I do calm sitting." Calm sitting is modeled and practiced. You need to identify clear physical boundaries, such as a planned seating arrangement in school or a planned play area at home. Use consistent materials that are clearly marked and accessible, like toys that

are within easy reach and stored in or right by the area they will be used in.

In addition, expectations, such as the rules, rewards, and consequences, should be visually available. Once again, these must be clearly described to your child. After this has been completed, use charts with stickers or stars to keep track of reward systems. Use the letters of your child's name placed on a chart to keep track of consequences. Throughout the day, if letters have been received, they can slowly be erased for positive responding. This provides a wonderful visual response for appropriate behaviors, and you can deliver this feedback, depending on your child's needs, every ten minutes, fifteen minutes . . . three hours—you decide what works best.

INTERPERSONAL ENVIRONMENT

Second, your relationship with your child must also be consistent in both word and action. He must see you as a predictable person, a person in control, a calm person, and, finally, a person who keeps his word. Being "easy" or giving your child a "break" will hinder your effectiveness. You make rules and stick to them. You make requests and follow through; you don't make second requests, and you don't plead. Your interactions must be stable, allowing your child to anticipate how he will respond. He must see you as someone who can help him understand the world around him. The highest praise I can receive from a child is being thought of as his helper or problem solver—"Ask Mrs. Grayson, she knows how to help." "Mrs. Grayson is a problem solver." "Did you know Mrs. Grayson's job is to help me figure things out?" If you are only seen as a problem causer, your effectiveness will be minimal. You must be highly organized and pay attention to details as you create a structured environment for your child. However, you must be able to remain flexible within this structure. By doing so, you will provide the structure your child needs to learn to be flexible.

REINFORCERS

Third, reinforcers will need to be very individualized, as the Asperger child or teen often does not respond to typical reinforcers. You must be well aware of what your child views as a reward. Incorporating obsessions into a reinforcement system is an appropriate way of offering a strong reinforcer and of also controlling access to an obsession. You need to make sure your child is aware of how the reward/consequence system works. Natural consequences can also be highly effective and will remove the "giving" or "denying" of the reward from you. An example of a natural consequence is: "If you finish your morning routine within a certain time limits you will have time to watch a favorite TV show before school. If you take too long, you will not be able to watch the show." Favored activities should follow less favored or challenging activities. A word of caution: reinforcers can also cause difficulties if they are used too frequently. Not only will they lose some of their potency, but struggles can arise over the giving or not giving of the reward.

DAILY ROUTINE

Fourth, at both home and in school, develop a daily routine so that your child knows what he is doing and when. Posting the schedule and reviewing it when your child becomes "stuck" can provide the necessary prompt to move on. In addition, compliance is not a struggle between you and your child, but rather simply a matter of following the schedule. The individual views the schedule as a guide. As noted, a guide will always serve to decrease anxiety, which in turn decreases behavior issues. I have heard my students tell visitors who enter our classroom, "That's our schedule; don't erase it or we won't know what to do." This is said even by students with excellent memories, who from the first week of school could perfectly recite the daily schedule for each day of the week (again, during sabotage, a goal will be to decrease the importance of the schedule as the year progresses).

The important detail is to review the schedule. We have seen many situations where detailed schedules are written, but never regularly and carefully reviewed with the child. As you review the schedule, you not only lessen anxiety, but you also provide an opportunity to discuss appropriate responding. When you develop a schedule at home, you may number the items on it, such as 1, 2, 3, but try to avoid assigning times to each event or activity. It is often difficult to do things to the minute, and failure to do so can lead to further upset for an Asperger child. You may also choose to establish a routine for only a small portion of the day, if you feel a day-long schedule would be too great a change for your child. For example, you might create a schedule for an activity, such as going to the mall, as an easier place to start. For a teen, rather than using a written schedule, you could use a desk calendar or day planner. Again, this accomplishes the goal of providing a visual guide. We will discuss the use of schedules in greater detail later on in this chapter.

The creation of this environment will take time and will require you to examine more details than you knew existed in any environment. Your reward, however, will be the miracle of watching your child leave his anxieties and problematic behaviors behind. You will see him begin to really trust you and take chances he never thought he could. You will witness his gradual and steady steps into a larger world.

Using Language

It's time to expand your ideas of how to use language and to explore how you can use it as a powerful tool to decrease anxiety and increase compliance. Remember, gain your child's attention before you begin to speak. You should be physically close to him (though not in his personal space) and, for the young child, on his eye level. Your language should convey meaning, provide the "road map" or "game plan," and enable your child to respond more appropriately. These children don't have the road map we all have and take for granted, which allows us to maneuver in the world around us. Language used in a concrete, predictable manner becomes a way to teach alternative behaviors. For example, even after social skills training, saying to Max, age nine, "Today after school, Mom is taking you to the playground to make and play with a new friend," doesn't provide enough information. He doesn't know what that means or what is expected of him. Instead, I would provide Max with the following "game plan."

"HOW TO MAKE FRIENDS"

MRS. G.: Today your job is to go to the playground to make a new friend. You will use the rules we learned for making a friend. What do you have to do first?

MAX: Look for a child my own age, go up to him, get his attention, and say, "Hi, my name is Max. What's your name?" He will tell me his name and I'll say, "Hi. Do you want to shoot baskets?"

MRS. G.: That's great. Max, it is also important to remember the rules for shooting baskets. Do you remember any of the rules?

MAX: I remember we take turns and we have to decide how many times we can shoot in a row. But how will we decide who goes first?

MRS. G.: Would you be okay letting the other child go first? Then you could ask him, "Is it okay if I pick how many shots we can do in a row?"

MAX: Yes, I can be okay with that.

MRS. G.: Remember, Max, you can pick one to four for how many shots you can take in a row. You can't pick more than that; it wouldn't make sense. Okay?

MAX: That's okay.

MRS. G.: You also have to decide where you will stand when you shoot baskets.

MAX: The playground has a shooting mark on the ground— I saw other kids use it. That would be fair.

MRS. G.: I agree with you, Max. That would be a good way to decide.

Notice above that I review the rules for shooting baskets, such as how to decide who will go first, how to take turns. Even if they have been discussed before, generalization won't occur without guidance. Remember, a problem planned for is a problem avoided.

We would also practice some simple scripts to be used in conversation. Developing language scripts to be used in novel social situations is a crucial element of any preparation technique.

MRS. G.: What could you and your new friend talk about?

Remember, conversations go back and forth. You will need to ask questions and make comments. Do you have any ideas?

MAX: I can tell him all about geography. You know I can name all the states and their capitals.

MRS. G.: Max, we talked about this before. The states are very interesting to you, but they are not interesting to other children. Other children would only talk about the states if they were doing a report for school or if they were going to a particular state to visit. You need to pick a topic that will be interesting to the person you are talking to. Can you think of anything a boy your age, shooting baskets, might be interested in?

MAX: I think he might be interested in sports.

MRS. G.: That's a great idea. Could you talk to him about basketball and other sports? What could you ask him?

MAX: I could ask him if he goes to basketball games, because then he would ask me, so I could tell him I go with my dad. Could I ask him his favorite team?

MRS. G.: Yes, that is a great question. Then you could tell him your favorite team. Also, when you are shooting baskets, make sure you comment on his shots with nice statements. Can you give me some examples?

MAX: "Good shot. I liked that shot." I could even say, "You can have another try" when he misses.

MRS. G.: Max, you have some great comments and questions. Just remember about going back and forth.

Notice I never just say, "Do this . . ." or accept yes/no answers. I make sure each step is clearly outlined and that Max tells me exactly what he will say or do. The above sequence may involve even more examples depending on the age, prior social experiences, and conversational skills of the particular child. Finally, we would work on a plan in case the first child rejects the play offer.

MRS. G.: Max, what would you do if the child you ask to play says no?

Max: I would ask again and again. Then he would play.

Mrs. G.: If you do that, the child will think you are a pest [it's good to have a previously decided keyword that illustrates a given type of behavior] and will never want to play with you. Remember, the rule is, if a child tells you they don't want to play, you have to walk away and find another child to ask. You can only ask a child once to play.

Now when Max goes to the playground to make a friend he has a plan to follow.

REFRAMING

When your child misinterprets a situation, your language can be used to reframe the situation, allowing your child to reinterpret it appropriately. This reframing can also be used when your child engages in inappropriate behaviors. Through your language, you provide alternative responses for the future. More important, your language can be used to introduce new ways of thinking or rethinking previously held beliefs.

An example of this would be the introduction of new foods into a child's repertoire. This was a goal for Mitch, an eleven-year-old who would eat very few foods. More disturbing, the particular foods he ate made him seem unusual to his middle school peers (the same soup brought from home each day, cold noodles, etc.). In beginning to work with Mitch, the idea of eating new foods was introduced by linking the eating of new foods with age-specific skills. The discussion began by asking him to recall different skills he had learned at different ages (crawl/walk/run, cry/sounds/words, drink from a bottle/sippy cup/regular cup, etc.). This led to the development of a new system to classify how a child changes: the preschool way, the elementary school way, the middle school way, the high school way. Trying, eating, and then incorporating new foods into his diet was put into this system with specific foods for each category. Items such as pizza, sandwiches, hot dogs, burgers—typical adolescent foods—were included in the middle school category. This language approach was paired with a step-by-step program to actually introduce the new foods. In addition, we helped Mitch to view eating these new foods in a different way (we reframed his approach to new foods).

"ACTING YOUR AGE"

MRS. G.: Mitch, are there things you can do now that you couldn't do when you were a baby?

MITCH: Oh yes, lots of things. I couldn't use the computer. Also, did you know I couldn't talk?

MRS. G.: Yes, that's true for all babies. I bet it is also true you couldn't walk or hold your own utensil when you ate.

MITCH: When you grow up you learn more things.

MRS. G.: You're right. That also happens at school. I call it "the preschool way," "the elementary school way," "the middle school way," and "the high school way." For instance, when you were in preschool you scribbled, but in elementary school you learned to color in the lines. When you were in preschool you had quiet time, but now in middle school you go out on the playground.

MITCH: You know what else? In preschool, and sometimes even in elementary school, I didn't raise my hand, but now in middle school I do. Now I know about interrupting.

MRS. G.: Well, there are other things, Mitch. In preschool you just had a snack at school. In elementary school you packed your lunch and you brought almost the very same food every day. In middle school, the rule is, you start trying different foods by buying your lunch. Students in middle school don't pack lunch every day. Do you like hot dogs? [I knew he did.]

MITCH: Yes, I do, but I never bought one at school.

MRS. G.: The school sells hot dogs every Tuesday, so that would be a good first day to buy your lunch, since we already know you like hot dogs.

A social story and cue card with "the middle school way" were also created. Initially, Mitch bought the school lunch only on Tuesdays. Once this went smoothly, we met again to choose the next new food to try. Providing him with the visual of a weekly lunch menu helped to lessen his anxiety. Every Friday we outlined what he would eat each day of the following week. We also wrote down on which days he would bring a packed lunch and on which days he would buy lunch and what he would buy. Initially, to allow Mitch some choice, he had complete control over his packed lunch.

After a new food had been introduced and accepted by Mitch for two weeks, another new food would be introduced the following week. The same pattern was repeated, unless he initiated a change (for instance, he wanted to try a new food sooner, which he sometimes did after success with the second new food). His middle school goal was to eventually buy school lunch three days a week and pack lunch two days a week. Once this was established, we began to work on the foods he brought from home. This task became quite simple, because buying lunch had generated many new and appropriate food choices for Mitch that he could also bring from home.

Throughout this period, "the middle school way" was mentioned as frequently as possible. Whenever Mitch did something new or was successful in any new area, I labeled it "the middle school way" and pointed out he could not have done this in elementary school. This intervention, though presented as a whole, had three distinct parts:

- A system was developed to pair eating new foods with a rule ("the middle school way").

- A gradual step-by-step approach was used to introduce the eating of new foods.

- A reframing of Mitch's thinking about new foods was reinforced at every opportunity.

KEY WORDS AND PHRASES

When using language to teach new responses, developing and writing the keywords or phrases to be used when introducing or generalizing these new concepts will be important. In the above example with Mitch, "the middle school way" was a keyword for behaving in an age-appropriate manner. By making the words and phrases visual, you guarantee both greater understanding and usage of the phrases. Remember, using the phrases, not simply writing them, makes them effective. The words or phrases can be developed by you or by your child. Unusual phrases, ads, or catchy sayings are often attractive and easy to remember. The first step is choosing the area you want to work on with your child. Then select (or have your child select) a word or phrase to be used as a quick reminder for appropriate responding. With use, the key word or phrase alone will convey the concept and what appropriate responding will look like. This will allow your child to generalize a skill more easily. When the phrase is used in a new situation, he will know what to do, because the phrase corresponds to the new behavior. After one has been mastered, add other phrases as needed. Below is a sample list of phrases we have found to be effective:

SAMPLE LIST OF KEY WORDS AND PHRASES

• *Off the topic* (said to the child when his response is not on the topic being discussed)

• *Say one thing* (when answering questions or discussing a topic with too much detail—this skill should be practiced)

• *In your head* (refers to statements that should not be said aloud, usually statements about a person's physical appearance or statements that would hurt another's feelings)

• *MYOB* ("mind your own business")

• *Good choices/bad choices* (this will be explained in chapter 8)

• *Problems and solutions* (refers to a technique used to either prevent a tantrum or assist the child in regaining control during a tantrum)

• *School sitting, school walking,* etc. (refers to a specific manner of doing something that has been demonstrated to the child previously).

• *Just do it* (refers to times when the child must quickly respond in a particular way without question; especially useful when the child is involved with peers or when returning to mainstream settings from special education)

- *The rule* (It is very helpful for the child to have appropriate responses described as the rule; it appeals to their sense of seeing the world in black and white. Often simply stating that a desired response is "the rule" brings immediate compliance.)

- *Drop the subject* (refers to talking on and on)

- *Stick up for yourself* (refers to the type of response the child must make when being teased or taken advantage of by others)

- *Keep your problems small* (used when the child's behaviors are just beginning to escalate in a negative way; serves as a reminder to maintain control)

- *Bumping* (refers to interrupting others when they are speaking)

- *Stretching the topic* (attempting to go off topic by trying to make your new topic—usually a special interest—appear related to the original topic)

- *Being okay* (getting yourself together to handle a situation)

- *Use your words* (controlling yourself by using words when you are upset or frustrated, rather than responding with a meltdown)

- *Get your control* (key phrase used during a crisis)

- *Switching/substitutions* (key words used to remind the child about being flexible)

- *Being flexible* (it is very important that this concept is taught early, even to a child as young as five—in my classroom this is as important as reading and math)

- *Making changes* (variation of the previous two above)

- *Eyes up here* (key phrase to help with attending and focusing)

- *This is a choice/This is not a choice*

- *That doesn't make sense* (used when the child says something that is inappropriate, for instance: fantasy talk, mislabeling another's or their own feelings, giving misinformation on a topic)

- *Don't be a "me first"* (used with those children who have an obsession about always being first: in line, when playing a game, being called on, etc.)

- *Conversations go back and forth* (used as a reminder when learning how to converse with others)

- *Respond quickly and quietly* (often referred to as Q *and* Q)

- *Looking and listening* (often referred to as L *and* L)

- *The preschool way, the elementary school way,* etc. (illustrated on pages 74–76)

- *Show me* (add the phrase for what you want the child to do)

- *Tell me what you have to do* (often used after giving directions)

- *Dealing with disappointments* (refers to what to do when something doesn't go the way we thought it would)

- *Personal space* (not hugging, touching, etc., others when it is not appropriate)

- *Thinking with your body* (learning to use your body to communicate)

- *Thinking with your eyes* (learning to use your eyes to communicate)

- *Lower/raise your volume* (to help the child to modulate voice volume; often paired with a hand signal)

- *The way* (used to let the child know that you don't like the tone of voice they are using; e.g., "Can you try another way of saying that?")

- *Salvage the rest of the day* (refers to not allowing a problem to ruin the rest of the day)

- *Kiss* ("keep it small and simple")

- *Don't get stuck* (refers to not allowing a problem to control you or stop you from moving on; this skill is taught)

What you say is important, but how you say it can be the difference between success and failure. Sometimes a calm, even voice is needed; other times, a more dramatic tone may be called for. When you change the tone of your voice, point it out to your child. He doesn't use varied tones of voice to convey different meanings. By pointing this out, you communicate your meaning and you increase his awareness of the importance of paying attention to vocal tone. This should also be done with facial expressions and body language—two other modalities Asperger children don't use when communicating to or processing communication from others. Vary your facial expressions and body language, and explain and show how it helps you to understand what others are saying. Below are illustrations of incorporating key words and phrases into your interventions.

EXAMPLE: "STICK UP FOR YOURSELF"

Many children with Asperger's syndrome have difficulty riding the bus to and from school each day. Again, parents need to prepare their child for situations that will occur on the bus. Let's look at eight-year-old Jordan's daily bus ride to and from school with other special needs students. One of the other students, Dylan, was also diagnosed with Asperger's syndrome, but his behaviors were quite different. Dylan was very verbal, would become quite loud when anxious or upset, and, at times, could also become physical. On the other hand, Jordan's response to anxiety would be to stop talking and possibly cry or attempt to escape/ignore the situation. In spite of this, they had developed a friendship on the bus and began playing simple "travel games" to pass the time (their bus ride was forty-five minutes long).

Unfortunately, Dylan became quite agitated when Jordan began winning the games they were playing (initially this wasn't a problem, as Dylan had been the one to teach the games and so he won them all at first). Whenever Jordon won, Dylan began to talk to Jordan in a very loud voice, make unkind statements, and push him while he was belted in his seat. Jordan allowed this to occur and, because he did not complain, it was not reported by the bus driver to his parents or teachers. Finally, after enduring another bus ride like this—with the addition of Dylan's feet on him for the entire ride—Jordan's response was to tell his parents, in tears, that he hated school and would never go again. (It is often quite difficult, even for a very verbal Asperger child, to clearly describe the sequence of a problematic situation.) One hour later, after much questioning and discussion, Jordan's parents discovered the real problem. (Remember, with the Asperger population you must always look beyond the obvious.) Besides the short-term solution of dealing with Dylan's inappropriate behaviors, Jordan needed to learn a long-term solution. He needed the skills to deal with similar situations that would inevitably occur in the future.

To accomplish this, I first outlined Jordan's problem to help him identify which of Dylan's behaviors were inappropriate and therefore required a response from him. I helped Jordan to understand he had to "stick up for himself." We then discussed "scripts": the words Jordan needed to say to Dylan when he behaved inappropriately. "I don't like that; stop it." "Back off." "Move out of my space." "I won't ever play the game again if this is how you act." Jordan practiced saying these lines. Next, we discussed "the way": how you say these lines with regard to voice tone/facial expression/body language when you are "sticking up for yourself." Jordan again practiced these lines, now changing his voice tone/facial expression/body language. To foster generalization, he was given opportunities to practice with another teacher and his fellow classmates throughout the day. Only after this clear and specific instruction was he ready to respond to Dylan on the bus.

When communicating with your child, always use clear and simple language. Tell him exactly what he can and cannot do; be very specific and include all details. Your language should provide the information needed for completing a task or responding in an appropriate manner. Use examples when speaking, not explanations. For instance: "This is how school sitting looks," or "This is how you greet a friend," or "The rule is _____ ." When giving directions, be very specific and give them in a step-by-step fashion.

In addition, check and verify your child's understanding. For example: "Tell me what you have to do," or "Show me what_____looks like," or "You're showing me_____."

EXAMPLE: "BEING FLEXIBLE"

When your child misinterprets a situation, you need to interrupt and reinterpret the situation, providing the appropriate verbal labeling of the event. You are presenting a new way of thinking and, at the same time, labeling inappropriate behaviors as such. For instance, if a difficult change for your child is going to occur, you will want to introduce the idea of flexibility as a positive response. Prior to the event, you would ask your child if he knew what flexibility was. Depending on his age and response, you would accept his definition or modify it. The goal of the lesson is for your child to learn to define flexibility as being able to cope with, to be okay with, to handle, or to accept changes when they occur. Flexibility is presented as a positive rule to live by; people want to be flexible. You should also point out the problems that occur when he is not flexible and how being rigid always leads to difficulties. When the change event actually occurs, you immediately label it as an opportunity to be flexible and demonstrate what an appropriate response would look like.

For example, Adam loved to build with Legos. This was his favorite recreational activity, and he was very talented. However, he was also a perfectionist and his creations had to be identical to those included in the directions. If a piece was missing, he would have an immediate meltdown or would throw away the entire set, refusing to use any of the pieces. Adam was seven, and the concept of flexibility was presented in this way:

"Adam, do you know what it means to be flexible?"

"I'm flexible," he replied. "I just don't like change."

"Well, that's interesting, because being flexible means you are interested in changes, like the changes you can make on the computer. It means you can make a substitution. A substitution means trying to do something in a different way—a different way, not better or worse." I then gave him examples of times I was flexible, especially instances in which my flexibility worked to his advantage (no homework on a holiday, extra computer time, giving two treats instead of one). Together we planned situations for him to be flexible in, starting with unimportant events and working up to the important event, Legos.

To achieve this, start by developing a hierarchy of change with your child. The lowest item on the hierarchy would have changes he would find easy to accept; as you move up the hierarchy, the changes would be those more difficult for him to accept. Simultaneous use of the key phrase "being okay" or a social story would be helpful. Adam's hierarchy, which he helped to develop, looked like this:

1. Building a Lego model with a color substitution.

2. Playing a board game and substituting different game pieces.

3. Completing a puzzle with two missing pieces.

4. Building a Lego model with two missing pieces.

5. Building a Lego model with three missing pieces.

6. Building a Connect model with multiple (more than four) missing pieces.

7. Building a Lego model with four missing pieces.

8. Building a Lego model with multiple (more than four) missing pieces.

Adam began by working on the first item on the hierarchy. After he had repeated this activity a few times, showing he could "be okay," we moved to the next level of the hierarchy. It is very important to successfully master a level before moving up to the next one on the hierarchy. In addition, it is equally important to incorporate the word "flexibility" into your daily language. Provide opportunities throughout the day for both you and your child to be flexible. Always point out these examples, giving praise for all instances of flexibility and showing him how flexibility caused events to go much better. In my classroom I have a "flexibility box," and a student's name is placed inside each time he or she shows flexibility at home or in school. Once a month a reward is given to the student whose name appears most frequently.

"Being flexible" can be used for any transition or resistance-to-change issues the child is having. In this way you are transforming an issue your child sees as negative, enabling him to look at it in a new, different, and more positive way. You are providing a plan for how he should respond and allowing him to practice those responses under your guidance.

Using Visuals

Children with Asperger's learn most successfully through visual modes. They are visual learners, as well as visual thinkers. Generally, areas of strength include word recognition, oral reading, spelling, and letter/number recognition—all areas requiring visual learning. Therefore, visuals become a crucial part of almost every prevention strategy. Visuals serve to enhance understanding when new concepts are presented. They do this by:

- Helping to focus attention

- Acting as a backup when new information is presented, giving the child something to look at in case information is forgotten or confused

- Providing external organization and structure, e.g., by showing the sequence or steps needed to complete a task

- Remaining stable over time, allowing the child the needed time to process and respond

- Making concepts more concrete, which also decreases anxiety

- Acting as cues when the child is ready to practice the concepts

Visuals come in all shapes, sizes, and forms. Below is a partial list.

assignment sheets	lists of rules	sequence cards
cartoon bubbles	masking tape	signs with key
checklists	photographs	words and
color coding	pictures	phrases
cue cards	planning sheets	social stories
drawings	problems and	timers
footprints	solutions sheets	words
hand signals	problem wheels	written scripts
highlighting	schedules	

Let's explore how these can be used. Tim, an eight-year-old, was experiencing great difficulty whenever he played with peers in his neighborhood. He had responded well at school to a high degree of structure, consistency, and specific recess rules presented in a visual format. He had been given a road map for recess success. However, this was not the case when he was playing with peers in the neighborhood. In this less structured setting, where he interacted with different children in multiple activities, he displayed many inappropriate behaviors. When he didn't know how to respond, or if he didn't like the response of another child, he would push or hit them.

My initial response was to complete, with Tim's help, a problems and solutions sheet (this technique is described in detail in chapter 8). First, we outlined his neighborhood playground problems to ensure that he understood what was occurring. Next, we discussed both appropriate and inappropriate ways to respond in these situations. This was done in a very clear, step-by-step fashion and, ultimately, became his "game plan" for neighborhood play. It included both the rewards for appropriate behaviors and the consequences for inappropriate behaviors, using naturally occurring rewards and consequences as much as possible. For instance, when you play appropriately, other children will want to play with you and will be less likely to tease you.

During this process with Tim, it became clear that even with reading the "game plan" right before he went out to play, he needed a visual available to him while he was actually outside. Since his common response was to push or hit with his hands, I decided to put a symbol on his hand. Again, this was discussed with Tim. It was presented like many of the other strategies, as something that would help him solve his problem. I explained that we'd use his right hand, because this was the hand he used for pushing or hitting. I allowed him to choose the color of the marker we would use and what symbol we would draw. He selected a purple star; this was placed on his hand every day before going out to play, at which time the problems and solutions sheet was also reviewed.

When Tim returned home the first time the purple star was used, he said, "It worked. I was going to push John and when I saw the star it made me stop." The power of visuals! Both the problems and solutions sheet and the purple star were used for three weeks. Beginning with the fourth week, the reading of the sheet before going out to play was eliminated, and the following week the star was discontinued. By then, Tim had internalized a new way of responding. Remember, this does not replace ongoing social skills training and helping Tim to expand/generalize his interactions with peers.

SCHEDULES

As noted earlier in this chapter, schedules can lessen anxiety and the resulting behavioral issues. They are another powerful visual we use to give structure to the child's life. I don't think you would ever find an Asperger classroom that did not post a daily schedule. These are also especially useful for those home environments in which the child attempts to be in control. In these cases, a daily schedule is developed that breaks the day into intervals of thirty or sixty minutes to account for all of the child's waking hours at home. Initially, you may feel more comfortable starting with a schedule for just one hour or one part of the day. That's fine. Start with this and, as your confidence grows, increase the time covered by the schedule. If you are comfortable with the idea of scheduling, you can plan for the whole day from the very start. Activities for each time period are carefully outlined. Nonpreferred activities are followed by preferred activities as a natural reward or consequence for compliance. The preferred activity is not allowed until the previous nonpreferred activity is completed appropriately.

Schedules are often needed at times when your child is experiencing multiple changes. I caution families who don't need to use schedules on a regular basis that certain events (the start of a new school year, the end of the school year, new parental job, new sibling, moving, sickness in the family, hosting a party, hosting overnight guests) will probably require a schedule to ensure a positive response. Schedules are also needed at home during less structured time periods, such as weekends and holidays. These times often have too few events and, therefore, less structure and predictability. A schedule adds the structure your child needs for his comfort.

As with other techniques, the schedule is developed with your child. When developing a schedule for a specific event, it should be developed in advance so that it can be reviewed multiple times before the event occurs. The schedule should be as specific as possible, but remember, to the Asperger child, "As it is written, so it is done." Asperger's children are very literal, so when developing a schedule, build in the possibility of change. For instance, driving to the mall may take twenty minutes, but it might take forty minutes. Or, remember you can pick one movie at the movie store, but your favorite may not be available. In addition to planning for the unexpected, you are also teaching flexibility. A sample schedule for overnight guests follows. But remember, while there are specific items on the schedule, you will need to have your child understand that these are approximate times. You will need to prepare your child for the possibility that each activity on the schedule may not be completed at the exact time shown on the schedule. While exact times can be followed on school schedules, this level of exactness will not be able to be used at home. This is an excellent opportunity to practice flexibility.

"COMPANY SCHEDULE"

8:00   WAKE UP AND DRESS (our guests will use the blue bathroom)

8:30   EAT BREAKFAST

9:00   PLAY WITH OUR GUESTS KATE AND BILL (remember the sharing rule)

10:00   GO TO MY SISTER'S SOCCER GAME (I can sit and cheer with my family and guests or play on the playground by the soccer field. Kate and Bill can also pick what they want to do. It is each child's choice.) [As is probably obvious by this addition and the earlier statement regarding which bathroom the guests will use, this child likes to control the situation and all the individuals in it. The schedule has to be developed with the child's special issues in mind.]

12:00   LUNCH AT OUR HOUSE (going to McDonald's is not a choice; deciding what I eat is a choice)

1:00   OUR COMPANY MAKES THE CHOICE: ZOO OR SCIENCE MUSEUM OR MALL [Including three choices, rather than leaving the choice completely open, will help relieve anxiety for the child.]

5:00   DINNER IN A RESTAURANT (I can pick between Friday's and Maria's)

7:00   VIDEO (Kate and Bill get to pick the video because I picked the restaurant) [As this child has eating issues, and likes many children's videos, it is prudent to allow him to control the restaurant choice (a difficult situation) and let him practice sharing control of the video choice (an easier situation).]

8:30   BATH AND BED (Remember Mom picks where all our guests sleep—this is a choice for parents) [By not saying where each guest will sleep, but only who will choose, it allows for some needed flexibility in this area. If the child has had a smooth day and enjoyed the other children, you might permit the children to sleep together. You now have an opportunity for the child to practice a much-needed and common social skill—the sleepover. If however, the child appears stressed or the day has been "bumpy," you can provide the child with the necessary privacy.]

As with schedules, the additional visuals below can also be used to provide visual cues for what to do and/or how to do it, thus fostering your child's understanding and independence. This approach makes the model more skill-centered, as opposed to prompt-centered.

CUE CARDS

The use of cue cards is especially effective when your child is in a mainstream school setting, in the community, or attending a social event, although it's also useful at home. A skill is first introduced, taught, and practiced with the child, and then a phrase or saying is developed as a shorthand means to remind him of the appropriate response. This is written on a small index card, which can be placed in a desk, a book, or pocket for easy reference.

HAND SIGNALS

Hand signals represent another form of visual cues. As with cue cards, they are a better choice for public or integrated settings. When a child is having difficulty, a hand signal, chosen by the child and the adult, can be used to privately signal the child to change or stop a particular behavior. For example, Jack, an eleven-year-old, had just joined a Boy Scout troop with his peers, without support. While he was able to complete the troop activities independently, he had difficulty answering questions—his answers would go on and on. Using a signal, his troop leader was able to limit his answers. When Jack continued talking after giving a sufficient answer, the leader would place his hand on his shoulder as a cue. Since Jack always sat near the leader (usually the best seating for an Asperger child), this was not a problem, nor was it at all obvious to his peers.

Ellen, a twelve-year-old, enjoyed going to the mall, but often flapped her hands because she was excited. The hand signal her parents settled upon was snapping their fingers. This signal served two purposes: it made Ellen aware of her hand flapping and it reminded her to stop.

SEQUENCE CARDS AND CHECKLISTS

When learning a new skill or completing different tasks or activities, the Asperger child can become quite anxious. This can be the result of:

- The introduction of novelty (never a favorite among those with Asperger's syndrome)

- The feeling that the task will somehow interfere with an established ritual or obsession

- Not knowing exactly what to do

- The concern that they may not complete the task perfectly or the realization they won't be able to complete the task perfectly

This can often lead to an inappropriate response on your child's part (e.g., verbal arguing, noncompliance, a tantrum). By providing step-by-step sequence cards or a checklist of steps prior to introducing a task or activity, most of this can be avoided. Cards and/or checklists can be used for dressing, grooming, morning/night routines, homework, or almost any academic task.

Drew, a seven-year-old, found drawing difficult, especially when asked to create his own picture. He simply did not know how to start and would immediately become anxious. The following sequence card was developed and used prior to his completing a homework assignment. Similar cards were used for additional drawing activities, each with fewer directions, until they could be discontinued altogether. An example of a sequence card to teach game-playing skills has also been included below.

"HALLOWEEN PICTURES"

You are going to draw a picture of a pumpkin. You will also draw a picture of yourself. There must be two things in your picture: a pumpkin and you. [Here you clearly state what will be in the picture.]

When I draw:
1. What will I draw?

2. What will be in my picture? [Again you are assisting the child in knowing exactly what they will be drawing.]

3. What will I be wearing?

4. Where will I be?

5. Where will the pumpkin be?

Remember:

1. Before I draw I think of ideas. I might have to change some of my ideas, if they are too hard to draw. [Asperger children often will have very specific objects/people/animals in mind to draw, representations well beyond their skill level. This needs to be discussed and decided upon before starting the picture.]

2. When I am ready to draw I use a pencil first, so I can erase.

3. When I am all finished drawing with my pencil, I can start to color my picture. [This direction allows for mistakes to be easily erased.]

4. When I color I use many different colors that make sense. [This direction avoids having the child use only one color or colors that are not appropriate; often Asperger children have an obsession with a particular color.]

"HOW TO PLAY A GAME"

Below is an example of a sequence card to teach game-playing skills.

1. Pick a game to play [The child selects three or four age-appropriate games, which are popular and can be played with others.]

2. Learn the rules:

   a. Where to start

   b. Where to end

   c. How to move

   d. What to touch

   e. What to do when you move [The child must clearly know how to play the selected game.]

3. Ask someone to play:

   a. "Would you like to play _____ ?" or "Do you want to play _____ ?"

4. When you play:

    a. Follow the game rules.

    b. Decide who goes first.

    c. Take turns.

    d. Ask for help if you don't know how to play.

    e. Wait your turn.

    f. Touch only your own game piece.

    g. Make nice comments, like "You can go first." "Good try." "Don't worry, you'll get another turn." "I can show you how to do it." [Additional sentences or a more comprehensive script may need to be developed, depending on the age/level of the child and on the particular game selected.]

5. Playing is fun. Sometimes you lose and sometimes you win. You are always a good sport. Good sports say, "Good job!" "I had fun." "Congratulations!" [If winning and losing have not been previously discussed with this child, it should be done prior to game playing. Losing is usually a difficult area for the Asperger child. A social story addressing winning and losing, combined with practice before playing a game with peers, is often needed.]

TALKING WHEEL AND VOLUME CONTROL

Anything you can use to make a task or skill more visual will lessen anxiety and foster comprehension and learning. Children with Asperger's syndrome are often unable to control the volume of their voice. Visuals can also be developed to assist in this area.

A talking wheel is used to teach younger children about the different voices that can be used, depending on the circumstances. A large circle is divided into four quarters: silent, whisper, talking to another person, and talking to a whole group. The child practices each of these "voices." At the same time, a list of when each "voice" should be used is created.

Volume control refers to another visual. A thermometer is drawn on a piece of paper. At the top of the thermometer the word LOUD is placed, in the middle the word NORMAL, at the bottom the word QUIET. Again, each voice is practiced and a list is developed describing when each voice should be used. The child is told to "raise the volume" or "lower the volume" either verbally or with a hand cue (hand is slightly raised or slightly lowered). Over time, your child will learn to respond to the phrases "raise the volume" and "lower the volume" in multiple settings without the visuals. You could also create a dial with the words LOUD, NORMAL, and QUIET placed around the circle. An arrow would be attached. When introduced, this would be compared to the dial of a radio or TV.

Special Considerations for the Teenage Years

Many of the points that are discussed in this chapter will also apply to teenagers. Stabilization will be extremely important for this age group. Prevention of problems will surely be the order of the day. However, your ability to control things will be severely compromised by your teen. You will not easily be able to control his environment, but you can use reinforcers to help you. Teens do not like to be controlled in any case, and Asperger teens are no exception. Everything you say and do must be more age appropriate. You can use visuals such as schedules, but make sure they fit your teen's chronological age. You will use language much more than with a younger child. More reasoning and discussions will be needed. Less direction and more negotiating will be important. You may have to teach your teen how to have a conversation, especially about an unpleasant topic. Many Asperger teens will never have had a productive conversation with you before this point. Anticipation and future vision are quite important because the Asperger teen's emotions are usually much more intense than a younger child's. You do not want to be dealing with problems once they have exploded upon you and your teen is in the middle of a meltdown.

SOCIAL ISSUES

Whatever degree of ease or difficulty the younger child had socializing, the problems are greater as a teen. Arranging play dates or orchestrating and supervising social interactions is virtually impossible unless your child's teenage friends are those who also have special needs. If your teen has friends who are also atypical, you may be able to play a bigger role in his socializing. You can facilitate, plan, and coordinate arrangements with other parents who are in the same situation with their teen. Arrange for structured get-togethers such as the movies, bowling, and the like.

For the general population, it is expected that social gatherings will be planned by the teens themselves. Your teen has to be able to initiate interactions with others via face-to-face conversations, the telephone, e-mail, or instant messaging. He also must have similar interests in terms of conversational topics and things to do. For example, many teens want to hang out at the mall, play sports if a boy, or talk about beauty and boys if a girl. If your teen is still into Pokémon or Yu-Gi-Oh!, it may prove to be too wide a gap to bridge to be able to interact with a typical teen. Therefore, early on in the process of helping your child, before he becomes a teenager, you need to have him develop more age-appropriate interests and skills. His interests may not be the same as the majority of his peers, but they must be similar to a subgroup of peers. For example, many children and teens are into sports. Your child or teen will probably not be. If his interest is in drawing, this is not a social activity. It is one that he can engage in by himself. He will need to be interested in things such as acting, where he can join an amateur theater group.

By far the most difficult aspect of social interaction is initiating contact with others. There is no question that the Asperger teen will find it difficult to do this. To initiate a social event, your teen must have the opportunity to do it. Peers from school, religious groups, or Scouts can provide the opportunities for your teen to make a face-to-face connection with someone. While the telephone can be another means to communicate, it is a difficult and anxiety-producing skill for most of the Asperger population. Try to develop this skill when your teen is much younger and the urgency is less. E-mailing and instant-messaging are also used by many teens but tend to be employed much less by Asperger teens.

Once you have moved into the details of helping your teen reach out to others, you will realize the importance of the timeliness of talking or calling others for a social interaction. They often wait until the last minute to try to arrange something, and this often results in the other person being busy. Or they may find the courage to call someone only to find that he is not there. Make sure you have worked on this aspect of a call—leaving a message, asking when he will be in, and leaving your name and number for a return call.

The final piece of the contact includes the remaining details surrounding the future event—the day, the time, where it will take place, and transportation that may be needed. All of these aspects can ruin or prevent an interaction if not planned for and addressed before the attempted initiation occurs.

SEXUAL ISSUES

Many typical teens begin their sexual experiences and knowledge through their friends. They talk to others and learn the vocabulary of sex, as well as a good deal of information, which may or may not be accurate. The Asperger teen may know nothing of the "street vocabulary" or only know technical information about sex. He may not know it from the teenage viewpoint. As a result, the Asperger teen is often naive, easily taken advantage of, or clueless. He must know the lingo that teens use as well as understand what to do and what not do from a teen's point of view. Parents usually tell their Asperger teens too little information or make it too technical. The Asperger teen needs to know the "nitty-gritty" of sex, dating, and relationships with others. His parents are often the only ones whom he will be able to talk to about sex, since friends may be unavailable. If you cannot do it, the professional you are dealing with will need to do it.

Distortions and obsessions about sex are not unusual and will need to be addressed in a very frank and explicit manner. It would be naive not to realize that your Asperger teen is a sexual being. Whether you give him any information or not, he will begin to gather it without you. The Internet has become a major source of information for everyone about anything they might be interested in, including sex.

Let's look at an example where no one told Sam, a thirteen-year-old, about girls. It seems that Sam liked a girl in his class. She, in turn, talked to him and appeared friendly. This platonic, innocent relationship continued for a month or two until one day Sam told her that he loved her. She became quite upset and did not want to be friends with him anymore. Sam, however, was not put off by her rejection, but instead began to follow her around the school each day, watching her from afar. Finally, the school staff became aware of this and had to put an end to his behavior, but not before a terrible scene occurred at the school dance. Sam was in desperate need to know about relationships with girls. If only someone had told him before all of this happened.

Sex, in some form, is an issue that can become an obsession for the Asperger teen. Pornography, chat rooms, instant love affairs, or cyberdating can all become areas of fascination for your teen. Of course, mature, healthy sexual interest and fulfillment is something that, once again, will need to be taught to many with Asperger's.

It is not unusual for teens to be on the Internet and become involved with chat rooms. When this occurs, it doesn't take too long before they move from chatting online with a person of the opposite sex to calling them on the phone. Boys are much more likely to do this than girls are. It is important to talk about relationships and "how they work" before something like this occurs. As always, anticipation and preparation are crucial.

EMOTIONAL ISSUES

Asperger teens will often be more immature than their typical age counterparts. Their interests, sophistication, and sensibilities will lag behind their peers. At times they may act much more like adults than like their peers; they will scoff at the immaturity of their peers, finding them too childish to deal with. Unfortunately, this only serves to distance them further from their age mates, leaving them with no chance to develop social relations with other teens. Do not let their intellectual, serious side pass as maturity. It is more of a pseudosophistication that masks substantial naïveté.

MEDICATION ISSUES
As your child becomes older, the need for medication often increases. The vast majority of Asperger teens will wind up on medications for many reasons: lack of early treatment, the increase in emotional issues with age, and the failure to develop and/or use coping skills.

ISSUES REGARDING LIFE AFTER HIGH SCHOOL
Many Asperger teens may graduate from high school but never go to college, even if they have been accepted. Or, if they go, they may drop out after the first semester. Your teen needs to develop the skills necessary to survive in a less structured environment such as college. They need to learn how to manage their affairs—being independent and accomplishing what is necessary for their school survival. If the Asperger teen does not go to college, what will she do in the world of work? Many do not work, some will have jobs requiring minimal skills, and many will get fired from the jobs they have because they don't understand the unwritten rules of the workplace. It is very difficult for the Asperger teen to find a job, let alone keep it. When she is hired, no one tells her about the unwritten rules of working, such as needing to listen to your boss, not bringing laser pens in to work, avoiding political discussions with customers, or opening packages with your teeth in front of customers. All of these things can, and probably will, result in being fired.

For example, Steve, a sixteen-year-old, obtained a job working in the warehouse of a chain store. He often had some downtime during his workday and needed to fill it with some activity. Not really knowing what to do, he brought in a laser pen. As he played with it in the storeroom, he spied a coworker climbing a ladder to retrieve a box. He turned on the pen, directed its beam in her direction, startling her, and she fell off the ladder. That was the last day he worked for that company.

Jobs that entail working with the public are the most difficult. All jobs have a social aspect to some degree—listening to your boss and cooperation with coworkers. All jobs have "work habits" as an essential component—showing up on time, taking appropriate-length breaks, doing your job well, following directions, accepting criticism, managing anxiety, being flexible, controlling emotions and obsessions, and so on. These are among the many skills you will need to develop in your teen—that should be started many years earlier.

At this point you have gained some understanding of the Asperger world and the different factors that affect your child. Take a moment now (and from time to time in the future) to reflect upon how the world feels and looks through the eyes of your child. Think about his behavior and the reasons behind it. Does he fit into any of the subtypes? Consider what materials you may need to work best with your child. All of this will help you to better understand your child and what you need to do. If you have done this, you are ready for the next chapter, in which we explain how to begin implementing these strategies and how to become an effective influence when working with your child.

5

Teaching New Skills

"It's How You Play the Game"

In the last chapter we discussed stability through structure and predictability. Now we are ready to teach new skills. These skills may replace inappropriate behaviors, or they may be new behaviors for your child. In either case, your child needs to learn how to do things as the rest of the world does them.

If You're Not Part of the Solution, You're Part of the Problem

As the parent of a child or teen with Asperger's, you need to become your child's advocate and an expert in what he needs. Become as knowledgeable as you can about the syndrome and the way your child displays the various symptoms. You also need to be the primary change agent. You need to be the one to help him develop the skills that will be necessary for his future. Schools tend to focus on academics. Many Asperger children have fairly well-developed academic skills. It will be the cognitive, behavioral, social, and emotional issues that will be the most important ones for your child to learn. You will be your child's most important teacher because you spend more time with him than anyone else and, also, because he needs to demonstrate the appropriate skills in the real world, not just in a classroom.

"I Think, Therefore I Am"

The approach we advocate assumes that your child is a thinking person. Just using positive and negative consequences are not sufficient for teaching new skills. We firmly believe that the Asperger child needs to learn new skills and understand their importance. He needs to develop an understanding of how the world works—what we do, when we do it, how we do it, and why we do it—for many situations that we take for granted. Your child does not know what to do, does not learn it through observation, and does not have an intuitive sense about what is right or wrong. You will be his teacher. There are two components to imparting new skills: the teaching techniques and the skills themselves. We'll discuss both in this chapter.

How to Teach New Skills

When working with your child, you must become the boss, the rule maker—a "sphere of influence." This is someone who has the power to make things happen. It does not always mean you will give him orders and he will follow them. Rather, you need to be the type of person who can exert influence in a situation to achieve appropriate results. You are a person who has the answers for every problem your child needs to solve. You are the problem *solver*, not just the problem *causer*. You will need to be this type of person in order to use many of the techniques and strategies in this book. This doesn't mean that you are in a power struggle. Instead, you engage in interventions that are effective and efficient and do not cause additional harm.

When you are trying to deal with any situation, you need to be the one in control. By being in control, you will reduce your child's anxiety, obtain compliance, and expand his repertoire. As his repertoire expands, he will also become more normalized, and, as an added bonus, he will have greater freedom from the rules that bind him. And in the end he will be a happier person.

We all know that, as a parent, being in control is not as easy as it sounds. If you are not in control, you need to learn how to be. To be in control, you always begin with small situations. Those that are small are much more manageable. Never choose the big battles to start with. Always begin with small events. However, one person's small situation is another's major disaster. Choose something that does not usually result in a major upset.

For example, where to do homework or pushing in the chair after getting up from the table may sound minor, but they may be good-sized situations with which to start. Begin with one and work through all the details, refining it as you go along. Never pick situations where there is a time factor or when you are in a hurry. Always remain calm but persistent in your direction about what needs to be done. Your child must also be calm when you are doing this. That is why you always give directions before the event occurs. After completing many of these small successes, you can begin to move to events that are slightly bigger, but still discuss them prior to an event and always in a calm and direct manner. It is important to realize that your attempts at being the boss will vary according to the age of your child. What works for a five-year-old won't work with a ten-year-old.

Here is an example: Billy, a seven-year-old, shows many of the typical behaviors we may see. He is a bit impulsive and anxious. Waiting his turn is not a favorite activity, so when he comes into my office waiting room for the first time and finds my office door open, he just walks right into my office. This becomes a small situation that I will use to become the boss. I ask him to come out into the waiting room with me and sit in a chair that I have designated. This is done in a direct but relaxed manner. Billy comes out and sits in the chair I have selected. I sit down next to him and ask him if he has ever heard of "office etiquette." He says no, and I begin to explain to him what it is.

"When you come into my office you are supposed to sit in a seat and wait for me to come out for you. You read a book or magazine, play with something you brought with you, or just sit and wait. Then I will come out of my office and say, 'Hi, Billy. How are you?' You will say, 'I'm fine. How are you, Dr. Sohn?' I'll say, 'I'm fine, too.' You'll then ask me if I'm ready for you. When I say I am, you can come into my office. Let's try it."

He says okay and I go into my office and come back out and we reenact the above scenario, prompting him where necessary. This scene is repeated, each time I see him, usually without much further need for prompting. I call it "office etiquette" as my shorthand way to communicate to him what he needs to do and also as a way for him to generalize this to other situations by just mentioning the phrase. Notice that I gave him very specific directions about what to say and do and then we practiced it until it was done right. Sometimes I've had to practice it two or three times to make sure it was done right. If I had accepted his incorrect completion of the task it would not have helped him get it right a week later when I saw him. I have given him new behaviors to replace the old ones and have subtly let him know that I am going to be the rule maker. I have also introduced some flexibility into his behavior since he has always entered others' offices in the same manner. Finally, because the issue was so small, it never became a battle.

Dealing with Teens

However, when you are dealing with preteens or teens, being a sphere of influence is somewhat different. As with all children this age, you will not have nearly as much power as you would like, no matter how much you try. With this age, you need to appear less authoritative, provide more choices, and develop skills in compromising and negotiation. More discussions are necessary. More patience combined with firm limits is ideal. You can still use many of the ideas that were discussed above, but make sure that you match them to your child's age—chronological and emotional. For example, John was a fourteen-year-old who constantly battled with his parents over how much time he could spend on the computer or video games. It was difficult to work this out because he was less willing to accept his parents' authority, as most teens are. We had discussions, using the methods that will be covered in this chapter, during which he slowly learned how to talk to his parents without fighting. He also learned to appreciate their reasons for wanting to curtail the amount of his computer time and became more interested in compromising and negotiating an agreement that was a win-win situation for everyone. In the process, his parents had to also accept the idea that they could not easily enforce the rules as they once had when he was younger. In the end he came up with an alternative activity that was acceptable to them and everyone was happy.

How to Change Thinking

In all discussions with an individual about a situation, there will be two aspects: 1) the selling of an idea (your part); and 2) the buying of an idea (your child's role). Both parts must always be considered together. The best "sales pitch" is incomplete if the new idea is not accepted, or "bought." This process requires constant monitoring of progress by the "salesperson," who should look and ask for feedback from the "buyer" regarding this step-by-step approach. A cardinal rule is to never move ahead to the next step without checking to see if the "buyer" is moving with you. If he is not, repeat the last step in another way.

For your child, this means that you need to convince him that there is a better way to look at and react to a situation than what he has shown you. He needs to hear what you are saying, maybe even see it, and then accept it if a better behavior is to occur. But you must realize that new thinking cannot occur easily, because your child is not a blank slate. He already has competitive versions of your idea. Different stories and interpretations are present in him that will compete with your new story or mindset. If the new mindset or thinking is to succeed, it must replace, suppress, complement, or outweigh every other story or competing version or idea. Only the most powerful argument will win out. Your prior history with your child is a very powerful force in this equation. All previous unproductive discussions and interventions that you have had with him will make your job that much harder, and must be replaced as well. To deal with these factors, you must be persistent, stick to the point, not allow irrelevant items to be brought into the conversation, and, finally, provide the reasons for the new thinking.

This is the time that you are making the implicit become explicit. By this I mean explaining what we do when something doesn't go the way we want or how we act when we don't want to do something. It is making things obvious that are not obvious to your child. You are laying out the steps to understand and solve a problem and having a discussion about it. You are explaining how the world works and trying to understand how he sees things. It's called "having a discussion."

Having a Discussion

Your discussion will rely heavily on the use of language. However, not all language is the same. You need to be very clear and precise in your word usage. Incorporating advanced vocabulary, word-based humor, and examples will help. The structure of the conversation is also filled with many examples, selected exaggeration, and emphasis on the use of nonverbal components as well, such as facial expressions and hand gestures.

This process begins with a conversation or discussion that is used to create new thinking and a new mindset, and it is absolutely necessary before a change in behavior will occur. However, there are many children and teens who do not want to have a discussion about upsetting events. For them, the retelling or talking about a troublesome situation means reliving it. They will say, "I survived the problem. I don't want to also have to talk about it." You must go slowly with these individuals and convince them how beneficial it will be for them to talk about it and learn from it. You must also not allow them to become too upset in the discussion.

Once you begin the discussion, your words must create a visual image. This image is able to communicate the desired course of action by creating a context that contains all the elements of the change—thoughts, feelings, and behavior. This is accomplished by attaching a phrase to this discussion that will convey these ideas whenever it is uttered. Such a phrase carries all of this information. Upon hearing it, your child remembers the conversation, the actions and thoughts it referred to, and then his new actions and thoughts. It becomes a shorthand version of the entire discussion and reduces the need for another lengthy discussion. In this process, you indicate verbally, as a list or so-cial story, all the issues that pertain to the topic at hand. If you are deal-ing with homework, for instance, the discussion would take place *before* the homework begins and might include things like where to sit, how long to spend on homework, how much help will be available, how to seek that help, what order to do the homework in, how to cooperate, other behaviors that are appropriate, and behaviors you don't want to see. Remember, having the discussion before the troublesome event is crucial. To do this you must be one step ahead of the problem, not one step behind. You must anticipate what has probably already occurred numerous times. It shouldn't be a surprise to you that a problem will oc-cur if it has occurred many times before. Unfortunately, you can become distracted and be thinking about something else at the moment that you need to be in the here and now. If you have too many other things on your mind you won't see what is coming until it is already occurring, and now you're one step behind. Don't keep hoping that it won't hap-pen. Deal with it as if its occurrence is a certainty.

For example, Mike had the same problem a number of times and we wanted it not to occur again. Rather than talk to him about it after the difficulty, we had a conversation about what to do the next time. Mike was a twelve-year-old who easily became physical with his peers when something did not occur as he desired. He needed to deal with this upset in another way, which we discussed. But to make this point really hit home, I talked about what he usually did and what he needed to do instead in a dramatic and emphatic manner with accompanying hand gestures. It went something like this: "Mike, when you're upset you literally and figuratively want to grab that other person by the shirt, shake him back and forth, up and down, smack him across the face, and throw him out the window. But that's not what we need to do when something is not going the way we want. Instead we need to let the problem slide away, like water off a duck's back. Just move on, don't get stuck, keep it small, roll with the punches." I said these lines three to four times to him. Each time he smiled more, then he began to laugh and repeat my words and gestures along with me. I had made my point in a dramatic, nonlecturing manner. In later sessions, his mother told me how he often repeated these lines during the week for himself and his brothers if they became stuck.

Selling the Real World

It is often necessary to have a discussion to help the Asperger child recognize and support our desire for him to be in the real world. To one extent or another, all Asperger children attempt to minimize their involvement with the world around them. We begin such a discussion as this by giving many examples to illustrate his fantasy world, such as phrases that he uses, facial expressions, and gestures. For example, he may stare into space or move his hand as if it's a rocket ship. This tells us he's not in the real world. We also discuss what it looks like to be in the real world. When we do this, we tell him that he should be looking at others, thinking about what is being discussed and stay on topic. Being in the real world includes awareness of others, topics of discussion, and body language. As the discussion moves on, we see if the child can distinguish between the two, as we provide numerous examples such as talking about something out of context or unrelated to the topic at hand. We then emphasize the need to be in the real world and the disadvantages of being in fantasyland. We list the advantages and disadvantages of each. If you are in fantasyland you won't know what is going on; it is harder to make friends since, others may think you are strange. In the real world, you can join in with others, learn new things, and have fun. Once the child has accepted these considerations, we ask them to begin to monitor their status during the week—real or fantasy—and we discuss it the next time we talk.

Finding the "Middle Ground"

One of the primary areas of change you will need to focus on is obsessive-compulsive behaviors. Obstacles to changing these behaviors are often a lack of flexibility and a desire to engage in preferred activities only.

Your child needs to understand that "life is a balance." As mentioned previously, most Asperger children are black-and-white thinkers, and they see the world as divided into two categories: things they *love* (known as preferred activities) and things they *hate* (known as nonpreferred activities). Since there is no middle ground, there cannot be any activities that can be in the *like* or *so-so* category. As a result, if they are not doing something they love, they must be doing something they hate. Therefore, it makes the most sense to the Asperger individual to only engage in the things he loves, and so the obsessive-compulsive behavior occurs and he repeats the same events over and over. When you begin to discuss this middle ground, your child may have no frame of reference to understand what you are talking about. He must understand what it means to just *like* something. You can't tell him to just find things he likes. You have to guide him. To do this you might draw up lists of activities that fall into four categories—love, like, so-so, and hate. You put events and situations into each group with the help of your child. As you do this, he begins to see that there is a middle ground. After this step is thoroughly expanded and discussed, you move to the second concept: "you can't always get what you want," meaning that everyone fills their day with lots of different things from each category. You explain how this works for you and others in his life and how this is the way life works. This becomes another life lesson.

For example, Judy, an eleven-year-old, never wanted to do anything that she did not like, no matter who required or suggested it. If you could get her to do something she didn't like, she would whine and complain, dig her heels in, and require some fair degree of coercion. In one particular instance at school, she could choose either staying in her classroom and reading or going to chorus. Reading was a highly preferred activity for her and chorus was quite undesirable. She didn't like the songs they sang and she didn't like standing on the risers to sing. But getting her to go to chorus could achieve many goals: it would promote a new activity and expand her repertoire, it would increase her social interactions, and we would also be teaching her to do something she didn't like without it becoming a major issue. Finally, we would be improving our ability to be rule makers. It would be a win-win situation for everyone.

We began by discussing her objections to chorus and then talked about how we all have to do things that we don't like. Many examples were used from my life and those of her parents'. The conversation was filled with some exaggerations and humor. She seemed to understand how all of us are faced with these same kinds of decisions. We didn't move on to the next step until we had a sense that she had absorbed our discussion and agreed with what we had to say. When we were certain she was ready, we moved to the step of telling her how we are able to do things we don't really like. We brought all of this together by telling Judy that the way others are able to do the things they do not truly like is to "bite the bullet," meaning they did something they didn't really want to do. We talked about the meaning of "bite the bullet" and how someone does it. We said that when others have to do something undesirable, they tell themselves, "It's okay; it's not really so bad; I'll get to read at another time," and other such statements. These comments make you feel that it isn't such a terrible thing to do something new or different, and it might even turn out to be enjoyable. Sometimes we even write some of these thoughts on a card or we create a story about them. (These are some of the visual elements talked about in the last chapter that are often necessary and can be in many forms, such as pictures, prompt cards, or social stories.) When all of this was completed, we practiced our own version of chorus with Judy and me standing on chairs (our own risers) in my office singing "Home on the Range" (a song Judy did not like) to her parents. In the end, Judy thought it was okay and was willing to give it a try on Monday when she went to school. However, we added that she had to do this without any fussing and fuming, to which she also agreed. The parents reported the next week that she did it, and eventually wound up continuing chorus for the entire school year. When I asked her in June what she thought about chorus, her reply was that she never came to enjoy it, but it wasn't really all that bad. But that was all we ever wanted.

As you can see, we solve problems in our discussions by trying to recognize what new skill needs to be learned and what subskills make up that skill. We teach each subskill one step at a time by talking about it, giving examples, presenting a good argument for using it, and then practicing it.

Changing Course in Midstream

In a slightly different situation, yours may be a child who does not like to switch an activity before it is completed. This is a particular issue when he or she is engaging in a highly preferred activity such as a video game. Sometimes you can wait a minute or two. Sometimes you can't. Other times, the activity never really ends. In these cases you have to teach the skill of "changing course in midstream," that is, stopping something one is doing and doing something different. This skill, like any other, is something you introduce as a concept, then move to specific examples, and finally practice many times before your child must try it in the real world.

Many Asperger children and adolescents have difficulty ending an activity before it is completed or they are finished with it. It is easier for them if the next activity is a highly preferred activity, but if it is not, you will run the risk of refusal, being ignored, argument, or tantrums as you attempt to end something they are doing. Since you know that this happens frequently you should be proactive and discuss this issue before the next occurrence. Sit your child down and talk to him about what usually happens when you want an activity to end. Discuss what he does as well as what he should do. Point out how his choice not to end an activity easily results in problems, upset, and all-around misery for everyone, including him. On the other hand, if he can keep the problem small, make a good choice, and be flexible, the degree of upset is small and everyone is happy, especially your child, who really dislikes excessive emotion and upset. Remember, have this discussion prior to the beginning of the problem activity and do not let him engage in it until the discussion has gone well and you are feeling that he has understood and agreed with you about what he needs to do. If he has not agreed with you, he will probably not do what you want him to do.

Using Real-Life Rehearsals as Well as Role-Playing

After you have discussed a skill or have planned an intervention, you must practice what you want your child to do. Just talking about it is not sufficient. However, most practice is done as role-playing only. When you role-play, you rehearse a skill in a pretend situation, not one that is real-life. You will say, "Let's pretend you are . . ." This is a good first step, but many Asperger children and teens do not demonstrate their newly acquired skill in real-life situations. Real-life rehearsal must also occur for your child to become proficient in doing something new. You need to practice it in real situations that you plan.

For example, Bruce was a ten-year-old boy who easily became upset when situations did not go his way. It was likely he would become verbally and physically aggressive to some degree at these times. We talked about his behavior and the reasons for his upset, and convinced him that he needed to change his actions to those that were less harmful to himself and others. He accepted this with relative ease. We went further and talked about alternative/replacement behaviors. After a short period of time, it became obvious that he could now give all the correct answers about a problem he had—why he did it and what he should have done instead. Unfortunately, he did not always do it the way he described it. He still became upset and aggressive. We had role-played many situations, during which he did well. However, these situations always lacked the emotional impact of real life that caused him to go off track. To deal with this, we began to put him in small, well-planned difficulties in which he had to use his skill. We could stop it at any time and discuss what he had to do and then try it again. These were real-time situations with emotional impact and afforded him much more realistic practice than role-playing.

In another example, Brian, a twelve-year-old boy, was easily upset and became angry when his parents attempted to control his access to TV. After discussing this numerous times and watching how he did with spontaneously occurring TV shutoffs, we decided to do some real-life practicing. With Brian present, we discussed with his mother how he had been reacting when the TV was shut off and decided he needed more practice rather than waiting for this event to occur naturally. I told both of them that I wanted his mother to randomly tell Brian she was shutting the TV off for varying lengths of time to help him become more flexible. Since he was already familiar with this idea and had practiced it in many other circumstances, he readily agreed that he needed to improve his ability to handle this better. His mother randomly turned off the TV during the week for different time periods, always letting him turn it on again later. In this way he became desensitized to the TV being turned off, realized it could be put back on later, and learned to accept his mother's action without much upset. It is very important to realize several important issues in this example:

• I had already become a sphere of influence with him, so he would readily listen to my suggestions. His mother was on the way to becoming an influence.

• We had discussed flexibility, good choices versus bad choices, keeping problems small, and avoiding upset and aggression because of the troubles they caused him.

• He had accepted the idea that he needed to be flexible and wanted to improve his ability to do so.

• He knew that we always practiced difficult tasks at home and my assignments were always seen as challenges for him to improve, rather than trouble we could be causing him.

• He always saw his parents and myself as allies in his struggle to be less aggressive and volatile. He knew we were trying to help him.

Without a high degree of certainty that these factors were in place, I never would have begun assigning him real-life practices at home.

Presenting Forced Choices

At times you may encounter great resistance to an initial change, and a strategy we use, forced choices, can make the first step possible. However, this approach should be used only when the above strategies have not succeeded, or when changing a behavior is critical (for instance, behaviors that are dangerous, interfere with health, or constantly interfere with your child's daily functioning).

It is important to remember that the Asperger child is often anxious and, as a result, attempts to control the world around him. The more control he can exert on his world, the less anxious he feels. Thus, providing choice in a situation allows your child to feel he has some control. Forced choices allow the following:

- Your child may choose between two choices/responses you have selected.

- You, not your child, have selected both possible choices/responses.

- Your child's completion of the task is not a choice, but selecting one of two ways to complete it is.

As with other strategies your initial introduction is crucial. Your child must feel as if he has a choice, but only a choice in terms of what you have offered. Make it clear to him that you know this task is very hard for him, but you are there to help him. However, make it equally clear you are not there to help him avoid completing the task.

Issues requiring the use of forced choice must be directly addressed to be resolved. By addressing a problem directly, you begin to teach your child alternative responses, not just for this issue, but also for other ones that have to do with being flexible versus being rigid. The prevention part of this strategy is your selection of a specific time to work on the issue. Although the issue may be occurring throughout the day, carefully choose a time to intervene (i.e., a time you can work individually with your child free of time constraints). Below is an example of using forced choices with a child who displays obsessive-compulsive behaviors related to task completion and perfectionism.

Sam, a seven-year-old, had many obsessive-compulsive behaviors centering upon the completion of fine motor tasks. These tasks, which permeated his day, had to be completed with certain materials in a perfect manner. Pencils had to be a certain length, sharp, and with a full, clean eraser. Crayons also had to be a certain length; broken crayons were to be especially avoided. When writing, no extra marks on the page were allowed and all letters had to be properly formed. In particular, the letters had to touch, but not go beyond, the lines. When coloring, the picture had to be totally covered, yet no crayon marks were allowed beyond the boundaries of the picture. Coloring had become especially problematic, because in order to ensure a picture was totally covered with color, Sam would go over and over the picture, pressing harder and harder with his crayons. Besides taking longer than others to complete a picture, he was constantly breaking crayons. Each time he broke a crayon (three to four per picture), he would become upset and demand a new, unbroken crayon. Not completing the picture was equally upsetting, so without a continuous supply of new crayons, a tantrum would result. At these times, his behavior was filled with rage. At home, he would destroy property and become physically aggressive toward his brother and parents. In school, he could no longer participate in mainstream activities involving fine motor tasks. Unfortunately, most school activities require this. After multiple approaches to change his behavior had failed, forced choice was used.

For Sam's first encounter with a forced choice, I selected a time we could be alone when I could remain with him for as long as necessary. I was well aware he would be unhappy with this situation and was prepared for resistance. Sam and I sat at a table with three crayons, a green broken crayon, a brown broken crayon, and a brown unbroken crayon. The worksheet I selected for him had a picture of a tree, which meant he had to use both the green and the brown crayon, because it was also important to him to color pictures with realistic colors. As soon as he sat down, he began to complain, "I need another green. This one is broken and I need green for the tree. I can't use this one."

I replied, "Sam, you have a choice. You can complete your work cooperatively and I will give you the unbroken brown crayon to use with the broken green crayon, or you can complete your work uncooperatively and I will give you the broken green and the broken brown crayon. These are your only two choices."

Sam began to verbally complain and attempted to throw the crayons. I immediately went into "crisis mode." I remained calm and repeated to him that he had a problem and I would help him solve it when he calmed down. Sam continued to complain, whine, and attempt to destroy materials for about fifteen minutes (in anticipation I had brought multiple copies of the worksheet, as well as multiple sets of crayons). At times, he would briefly calm down, but when the choice was restated, his behaviors would begin anew. During one of his calm periods, I was able to remind him we would be staying here until this activity was completed. He was immediately aware that this could result in missing his weekly checker game with a first-grade "buddy," a very favored activity (I had not picked this time to intervene by chance, being a strong believer in natural consequences). This time, Sam remained calm and asked me to explain "the conditions" (his words), again.

> MRS. G.: You have two choices, to use one broken and one unbroken crayon or to use two broken crayons. You need to show me you can be okay when you have to use a broken crayon. It's fine to want to use unbroken crayons, everyone does, but when a crayon breaks, the rule is: use the broken crayon unless the adult says it is too small.
>
> SAM: I can't. It's too hard to color with broken crayons. I can't do it.
>
> MRS. G.: That's why I'm here. I'm going to help you do it, because I know it's hard for you. Do you want to start with the broken brown or the broken green crayon?
>
> SAM: Can I start with the unbroken brown crayon?
>
> MRS. G.: No, you have to first show me you can be okay using the broken crayon and then I can let you use the unbroken crayon. Remember that's the rule.
>
> SAM: That's the rule about being okay with broken crayons?
>
> MRS. G.: Yes, it is. Can you be okay and show me you can use the broken green crayon to color the tree?
>
> SAM: Okay, I'm ready to color the tree with the broken green crayon.

It was necessary for Sam to verbally agree to "be okay," before he started to color with the broken green crayon. If he had not verbally agreed to "be okay," I knew his first attempt would definitely fail. As Sam began to color, he continued to verbalize how difficult this was for him. I remained by his side and responded in two ways to increase the likelihood of success. First, I acknowledged how difficult coloring with a broken crayon was for him and that I knew how hard he was trying. I also made sure to use many brief, positive phrases: "Nice work, Sam." "Wow, you are able to cover all the white even with the broken crayon." "Look, you are doing elementary school coloring even with the broken crayon."

Second, I provided practical advice for using a broken crayon. I did this by both describing and showing how to color with a broken crayon. This second step is critical. Remember, his fine motor issues were obsessive-compulsive, driven by a need to perfectly complete tasks. This need was rooted in anxiety. To change behavior, you must address the primary issue: in this case, anxiety. Showing and telling him how to color with broken crayons relieved his anxiety. In reframing the situation, I offered Sam alternative ways to color (switching gears or looking at a task in more than one way is quite difficult for the Asperger child) and provided the game plan for doing so.

Sam continued to color with the broken green crayon, with less and less verbal complaining as he colored. This reduction was due to the fact that he could now view coloring with a broken crayon as an option, because I had told and shown him how to do this. In addition, he was actually doing it and could see the visual results of his efforts—a very important step for a visual learner. As soon as he had completed the part of the picture that needed to be green, coloring it all using the broken crayon, we moved to the next step of a forced choice.

MRS. G.: Sam, you did great work! You colored nicely with the broken crayon, so you can do it. What do you think? Can you color nicely with a broken crayon?

SAM: Yes, but it is hard.

MRS. G.: I agree, and certainly if you had a broken and unbroken crayon, you would choose the unbroken crayon. But sometimes, you will only have a broken crayon and now you know what to do when that happens. Tomorrow, I can help you learn to color gentler and if you do, I think you will break fewer crayons, because I know you were having a problem with that.

Previously, I was unable to address this problem with Sam (pressing too hard) because he wasn't open to any changes with regard to his fine motor skills. Because of his success with an alternative behavior, he was now more open to trying other alternatives.

Our forced choice session was concluded in the following way:

> MRS. G.: Well, Sam, now that you showed me you can be okay coloring with a broken crayon, you can use the unbroken brown crayon to finish your picture of a tree. Also, because you were able to get control, there is still time left to play checkers with your first-grade buddy. You don't have as much time as usual, because you didn't get your control right away. Next time, if you can keep your control, you won't have to lose any time. I'm proud of the good choices you were able to make.

It was important to point out to Sam that losing control did have a natural consequence, but, because he regained control and completed the activity, there was also a natural reward. In addition, it was equally important to explain he was going to have less time with his first-grade buddy. Remember, these children always need a clear game plan before an activity begins, not once it has started. Prior knowledge will decrease the likelihood of future problems. And when they have learned these skills, we will teach them how to use them in other types of situations.

Conducting a Social Debriefing

"What just happened?" This is the process of reviewing what happened in a social situation. The event is reviewed in detail. Who did what and why, followed by the examination of options, better choices, and replacement behaviors. Incorporate as many of the previous ideas we have discussed to facilitate a new understanding of what occurred. Discuss and practice these ideas until they are incorporated into your child's repertoire. Do this following every unsuccessful and successful social situation. It is important for your child to know what went wrong, as well as what went right and why.

For example, an eight-year-old boy named Mark wanted to use his mother's umbrella one day to dance and sing on the sidewalk outside my office. He enjoyed this activity and since his mother had her umbrella that particular day, it seemed like a good idea to him. When his mother would not let him, he became angry and upset. When he and his mother finally appeared in my office, he was still upset and crying. He told me his side of the story and how he was angry with his mother. His mother told me how she was planning to let him do his song and dance on the way out of my office, but that had not satisfied him. She couldn't allow him to do it coming into my office because they were late for their appointment. My discussion began with a detailed listing of the events to clarify my understanding. I then told him that I thought it was not a good idea to do his routine either coming to my office or leaving it, whether time permitted or not. He looked at me in a disappointed manner as I explained further that there might be others who would see him do this. He replied that he did not care if anyone saw him. I asked him what others would think when they saw him and he was able to tell me they would probably think he was crazy, but he still did not care. It was good that he had some understanding of others' thoughts, but it was not complete. I asked him what others do when they think someone is crazy, but he did not know. I informed him it was possible they could tease him and asked him how he felt about that. Of course, he replied that he did not like to be teased. If he had told me he did not care about being teased, I would have pointed out how he has reacted in the past to such responses from others. We had to establish the idea that he did not want to be teased. I then told him that being teased is what happens when anyone acts in a peculiar manner, and my job was to help him avoid being teased. He immediately stopped crying and said, "If Mom had only told me that before, I wouldn't have been mad at her." We went one step further and talked about things he could do that would be fun that would not incur others' ridicule in any way. In this example, we helped improve "theory of mind" (an understanding of others' thinking) as well as engaged in a social debriefing.

Important New Skills to Learn

Many of the primary issues you will need to deal with involve issues related to anxiety, obsessive-compulsive behaviors, rules, tantrums, upset, and stress. Remember that the Asperger child is filled with anxiety, whether you see it or not. To relieve his anxiety, the child creates his own structure and rules. Routines, rituals and rules, and special interests give structure and predictability to what the child views as a chaotic world. The more your child can control the environment, the less anxiety he feels. However, even those who are masters of control will experience difficulties because they cannot control enough of what happens in the world. There will always be uncontrollable aspects that will cause distress. For this reason, you must help your child to overcome this control-tantrum cycle by teaching new behaviors that replace old, inappropriate ones.

You must directly teach your child skills to help him relieve anxiety and increase his flexibility. In direct teaching of a skill, you need to first rule out other alternatives that your child may be thinking about. For example, you might want him to do his homework, but he thinks he has a choice not to do it. No matter how many choices you might give him he will always have one more choice he likes better—not doing what you want but what he wants. He has to know that the option he wants is not a possibility at all. Then you need to point out the two choices he really has. Choice one is doing something a better way that you have outlined for him—the replacement behavior. Choice two is how he usually does this same activity. For both choices you point out what usually happens, making sure you include the negative behavior in detail. At this point, he should realize which is a better choice. If he has not realized how his normal actions are unproductive and harmful at this point, you have not sold him the new idea and he is not ready to discuss this further and in more detail. If he agrees with you about what needs to be done, he is ready and you can begin the more detailed discussion of what he is going to do.

Stress Management

One of the most important replacement behaviors involves dealing with upset. For each of us, there are many situations that cause distress, stress, and strain. When we can gain control over our emotions, we are in a better position to use our logic and reasoning to solve a problem. This is even more the case with the Asperger child. Almost any situation has the potential for upset. Many arguments, tantrums, and meltdowns begin with a trivial event. Some of these events have recurring themes to them, such as:

- Handling disappointments

- Dealing with unexpected events

- Making mistakes—not being perfect/"shades of gray"

- Blowing things out of proportion

- Dealing with rule changes

- Switching gears

- Ending a preferred activity

- Doing a nonpreferred activity

- Delayed gratification

- Getting stuck rather than moving on

To deal with these events your child needs to have skills that go beyond tantrums, rules, and rigidity. He needs to develop real *coping skills*. These are the ways that all of us deal with our problems. Most of these skills are not part of your child's repertoire, however. We will need to teach him stress resiliency, stress immunity, learned optimism, and "theory of mind."

STRESS RESILIENCY

This is the ability to bounce back from adversity and hold up under pressures and strain. "I get knocked down, but I get up again." As we get better at it, we are able to bounce back faster. For example, what may have taken an hour to get over now takes fifteen minutes.

STRESS IMMUNITY

"Like water off a duck's back." This is an extension of the above process to develop a longer-lasting solution to stress management. Once your child has learned some resiliency, keep helping him so that he can become more immune to the difficulties he may encounter.

The Asperger child tends to see only parts. He tends to see each situation as one that is unique. In order to learn from our problems, we must be able to make the connections between many different events and see the patterns that they present. This helps us to come up with solutions to our difficulties. Through repetition, explanation, and connecting the parts, your child can begin to see how pieces fit together and how they all make sense. Without a sense of meaning to an event, it remains a source of confusion, anxiety, and eventual upset. By joining the parts and helping the child to see how they are connected to other similar events, he can make sense of the world and develop prosocial skills. This will help him understand the real "rules of the world." This process is called *life lessons*.

For example, the TV is broken, cannot be readily fixed, and has become a source of upset. The child needs to be okay, calm down, and accept that there is little that can be done at the moment. The cable company needs time to fix the signal or the set needs a repair. However, the child usually feels that there is an immediate need for the set to be fixed. He has a favorite TV show that will be on very soon. He can't wait for it to be fixed, and wants someone to fix it right away, which is what usually happens with other problems in the house. There is now a crisis. A life lesson from a situation has two parts: 1) surviving or getting through the problem, and 2) the larger meaning that we can learn about similar situations. In this example, you will need to help him deal with the TV being broken and help him to learn that there are things that may break that cannot be immediately fixed. He also needs to understand that this happens and how it happens. Finally, he needs to understand why someone would not be able to fix it right away. In the end, the goal is for your child to be calm whenever any similar situation occurs. All of this is achieved through the discussions that were outlined above and the skills that follow. As you practice this with your child, you will realize which parts of it are the most difficult for him and see how to help him become more flexible and more resilient, eventually leading to greater immunity to problems when they occur.

LEARNED OPTIMISM

This is the ability to see the world in a positive light. Many Asperger children and teens can be quite negative. The slightest issue can be a problem for them. Sometimes no matter how much positive has occurred, they can only focus on what was negative. If they can see events in a more positive manner, they would be less pessimistic and therefore less anxious. They need to see that when things do not go exactly as planned or desired, it is not the end of the world. This is not just for one event, but it is something that applies to the broadest of areas—life itself. It fosters hope that "all is not lost" and is the crux of the discussion that takes place around a specific event before it is expanded to all of life's situations. We want to change the Asperger child's perception and interpretation of the events around him. Catch phrases that we want to insert into the discussion can include:

- *Next time things will be better.*
- *That wasn't so bad.*

- *It could be worse.*

- *I still got something I liked.*

- *It's not the end of the world.*

At times, during a discussion with your child, you may notice that any and all conversations only serve to perpetuate the negativity. In this case, optimism cannot be learned because pessimism reigns supreme. You will first need to end the pessimism by cutting it off immediately. I know this sounds arbitrary, but sometimes you will need to act like this. Your discussion isn't going anywhere and you need to help it move forward by changing its direction. Do not allow a negative discussion to continue. You can say, "We will not discuss this. You need to move on and not be stuck. I will wait for you to tell me you are ready to move on."

THEORY OF MIND AS A SKILL

"If I want you to know what I'm thinking, I'll tell you." The Asperger child's thinking process is often dysfunctional in that many of these children do not realize that other people have their own thoughts, plans, and points of view. They also appear to have difficulty understanding other people's beliefs, attitudes, and emotions. As a result, they may not be able to anticipate what others will say or do in various social situations. This has been termed as a lack of "theory of mind" or being "mindblind."

While this inability causes great difficulty, it may be possible to teach your child to at least appreciate or be aware that other people have different feelings, likes, and dislikes than he does. To achieve this goal you need to explain how people feel in many different situations. Do not just tell the child what to do, but help him to realize the reasons that others act in a certain way. See if he can tell you how he would feel in a certain situation. If his answer is reasonable, tell him that is how others feel as well. If his answer makes no sense or he gives one that is contrary to the general public, spell out the more typical feeling for him. However, discussion alone may not be sufficient. Pointing out feeling situations in TV shows or movies is often a good way to create a visual image to enhance his understanding. However, do not do too many at one time. This is a difficult concept and may only be learned in a rote manner and demonstrated infrequently.

Emotional Regulation

In order to handle our distress, it is necessary to control our emotions and not allow anxiety, depression, anger, and resistance to control us and prevent our use of logic and reason. If we cannot get past emotions, verbal strengths cannot be utilized. It is through our language that behavior control occurs. We use self-talk, as well as conversations with others, to make sense of what happens to us.

To understand emotions, we must distinguish between primary and secondary emotions. A primary emotion is what we feel first. The secondary emotion is what follows from it. For example, we feel anger (the secondary emotion), but the primary emotion that leads to this might be stress, a blocked need, or something else. If we understand the primary or underlying emotion we can figure out how to help. Thus, identifying these unmet emotional needs leads to a solution. For your child, anxiety is a major primary emotion that occurs for numerous reasons, but it almost always leads to a secondary emotion such as anger, upset, crying, or aggression. If we only respond to the secondary emotion, for example, the anger, we will miss the cause of the problem and no real solution will occur. If we respond to the anxiety, we will be able to address the real cause of the problem. Emotions must be understood and dealt with in a systematic manner, including the teaching of specific management skills.

ANXIETY MANAGEMENT

Anxiety cannot be measured or observed except through its behavioral manifestation—either verbal or nonverbal. A child can cry, complain of a stomachache or headache, crawl under the table, become argumentative, call others unkind names, or in some other way show distress. They may all be manifestations of anxiety. To manage the anxiety, we divide it into a number of parts:

1. You must recognize and identify the source of the anxiety.

2. You must help your child identify the source of the anxiety if she is old enough to understand this concept.

3. Make a list of numerous anxiety-producing situations, from easy ones to those that are more difficult (this is called anxiety mapping).

4. Create an anxiety hierarchy—put the events in order from easy to hard.

5. Prevent anxiety by external control—structuring the environment to make it predictable, consistent, and safe.

6. Gradually shift anxiety control to your child by preparing her for anxiety-producing situations by discussing antecedents, settings, triggers, and actions to take. She acts comfortable in these situations, and you'll know anxiety has been reduced when anxiety is no longer seen. If *not* calm, she asks for help and a further discussion ensues.

7. Further develop replacement behaviors and increasingly turn these over to your child to demonstrate. These alternative behaviors are the prosocial and appropriate complements to the inappropriate behaviors your child may currently demonstrate; for example, using words to discuss a problem instead of screaming.

8. Develop, practice, and rehearse new behaviors prior to exposure to the real situation.

9. Finally, implement new behaviors in the actual situations where anxiety occurs. Through your child's ability to demonstrate alternative behaviors and/or report being calm, we make the assumption that anxiety has been reduced.

10. If she is old enough, teach your child increasing independence in anticipating and coping with anxiety in a variety of situations.

This is the process used to determine what situations are upsetting. They will always start at the concrete level, but will quickly need to be expanded to other similar situations. For example, you may need to help your child learn to temporarily stop a video game. But at some point, you will have to extend this learning to the much broader concept of "switching gears," which means to end something before you are ready to do so. Your child must learn to do this in a variety of settings, using many of the skills and concepts we have already discussed—resiliency, structure, preparation, replacement behaviors, and so forth.

SELF-CALMING: BEING OKAY

As noted previously, one of the most important skills to learn is that of flexibility. It is the ability to cope with something unpleasant or undesirable. It is the ability to "be okay." This process requires no consequences, positive or negative, and therefore no external motivation, just good verbal skills.

As in all systems of change, you must have a good rapport and relationship with your child before you can introduce the concept of "being okay." If you are always arguing with him, if he sees you as a constant source of frustration, or if you are not a sphere of influence, it will be hard to succeed.

Achieving the first step of the change, accepting the idea of being okay, is the hardest part and takes the longest. Usually, this is a new idea for your child, and he may never have been okay before about anything, especially without a reward. So, you are attempting to integrate this concept into his thinking and have it become a part of his repertoire, but initially it is a completely foreign notion to him. It must first become an acceptable concept, but he does not want it to be. Therein lies the battle that you will encounter. It cannot be forced, but pressure will need to be used. You must strike the appropriate balance. As you work through an issue, you may find that greater pressure will be necessary. The Asperger child may feel that if he was okay one time, he does not have to do it again.

You may have difficulty with the first example or situation you use, and even the next one, until you have perfected your discussion and enough examples have occurred for your child to have integrated this concept into his thinking and he becomes willing to use it in some way.

Sometimes props, various objects, or activities are necessary to expedite the change. (This will be discussed shortly.)

Along with the concept of being okay comes the procedure you use to achieve this goal. You must "join" with him, talk the same language, and have him know that you understand how difficult this is. For the Asperger child, language is crucial. You must be concrete, explanatory, and use key phrases that are shorthand versions of difficult concepts.

Below is a step-by-step procedure for teaching your child how to "be okay."

Step 1: Introducing the Concept of Being Okay: Being okay means letting go of a problem or being able to do something different or new. It means the shrinking or minimizing of a problem, issue, situation, or concern. When we do this, we just move on; accept whatever it is and do it; or let it go and be done with it.

All of this is discussed in appropriate language, and never in the midst of a crisis. It is much more useful to discuss being okay about a future event, before it occurs. Problem situations are repetitive, and the particular problem you choose has probably occurred in the past and will occur again in the future in the exact, or a similar, form. You are trying to *prevent* the problem from occurring again.

Being okay can be used to do something new, stop doing something, change something, or respond positively to something. You must sell the concept of being okay to your child. The language you use is very important. The words must be concrete, clear, and precise. He will look for the loophole otherwise. Remember, your child does not really want to make this change and then be okay. He wants things to stay just as they are.

You begin by discussing how he has responded to a situation before, how his response created difficulties for him, and exactly what those difficulties were. They may include unhappiness, being upset, someone being angry with him, loss of an object or privilege, or being teased. This is the motivator or "hook" to be able to move forward. He must see being okay as a solution, something helpful, not as something problematic. Remember to point out that being flexible or okay usually means that a problem situation will go better or become smaller and that less upset will occur.

Your discussion about being okay involves a specific event or situation that requires a change in his behavior. You are first trying to achieve the cognitive change that is necessary before the behavioral component.

He must say "okay" after you have discussed the way in which he will make a small, concrete change. This increases the likelihood of its occurrence. A nod, grunt, or shrug is not the same as a full and complete "okay." You also discuss how our thoughts about something are as important as what we do. That is, how we think will determine how we feel and what we do. He must learn that he has it in his power to make himself feel miserable or okay. He needs to choose being okay.

You must determine the crucial "frame" or belief that makes it hard for him to be okay. Any of these beliefs will block your ability to move forward. For example, his "frame" may be:

- "Everything is very important to me."

- "I can't do what I'm told."

- "I'm scared."

- "I can lose and I must never lose."

- "Things must go my way."

- "I don't want to follow *your* rules, only *mine*."

He may introduce other issues that have nothing to do with the one you are discussing. He may do this to avoid the discussion or because he is unable to focus. In either case, ignore these issues and focus the conversation on the issue at hand, which at first is the content of the problem but then becomes the underlying thought process that is going on.

You must choose the correct words to "reframe" the problem so it has a more prosocial or positive definition to it. For example, some positive reframes are:

- "There are different degrees of importance."

- "I can decide to cooperate."

- "It's practice, not for real."

- "Make a good choice or decision."

- "I don't have to be perfect."

- "Newness and change can be fun."

- "I can try something new."

- "I can be okay with something new or different."

Being okay is discussed in terms of a small, but concrete, issue or situation. The issue may not even be the one you want to change, but rather a part of the situation, something much smaller that is more easily mastered and may be able to occur right away.

If the child is ready, he can actually try it out to see how it feels. Sometimes he wants to think about it before doing it. In that case, it may be necessary to put a time limit on how long he can think about it before trying it. You can help him try it by calling a first attempt a "practice" session, for example.

You will need to be persistent, but you must also know when to back off in trying to achieve the first step of accepting the idea of being okay, as well as the first attempt at doing something new or different.

A good amount of encouragement and support is needed. Also, the discussion can be done in a playful context, as if the change (being okay) is not a big deal at all. Or, it can be done in a straightforward manner, while still conveying the notion that being okay is not a difficult thing to do. Tailor the conversation to suit your child.

In order to enhance the acceptance of this new concept, it is often very helpful to once again point out the problems, difficulties, or other negative repercussions if he continues to not be okay with a change. Usually, these negative aspects occur as a result of others' reactions to him when he won't or can't be okay. You need to clearly explain this to him so he sees that not being okay has many unpleasant aspects to it. You may need to repeat this many times. You will point out how being okay will end the negative consequences and result in positive consequences instead.

You may need to give and discuss numerous examples, some in an exaggerated or even in a silly way. You should also discuss those behaviors he usually demonstrates instead of being okay, such as crying, yelling, running away, or refusing. Other times you will need to abandon the silliness and talk about it as if this is something very important that can even be helpful to him (as discussed above). In other words, you are tailoring your discussion to fit your child's way of incorporating information and skills into his repertoire.

For some, it would be appropriate to enhance being okay by giving a "high five," saying, "Way to go," or "You are getting closer to being the best boy in the galaxy," or something similar. Others do not need this, or even want it. Remember, you are looking for the most effective way to get this point across to *your* child. The technique itself does not stand alone. In other words, what he gains by being okay must be very important to him, and it needs to match your child's personality.

Being able to understand and access his worldview is a crucial factor in the change process. It may be necessary to repeat your first change again to see if being okay still holds for that first situation. Some particularly bright and clever children are able to be okay for something one time, telling themselves that it was a "one-shot deal." How they respond the second time will tell you if you need to do it again before moving to a new example.

Let's look at an example of how this works. Max is a seven-year-old who is very bright and verbal. An important issue for him is being the boss. He wants to be king and set all the rules in whatever situation he finds himself. He is also a "Logic Boy" who relies on his reasoning and logic skills to cope with the world. One day Max had a bad day at school. He was "shooting" his pencil at another boy in his class, despite the boy's plea to stop it. Max continued to ignore the boy's request until the teacher stepped in and told Max to stop. He refused and continued to aim his pencil at the boy and make shooting noises. The other boy continued to be upset, and Max was finally removed from the room. His mother told me her discussion with Max revealed he did this because his brain told him to do it and he could not stop. Needless to say, the mother was quite upset and thought her son was not only being disruptive in class, but was probably "hearing voices." My discussion with Max began with his retelling of the event, interspersed with my questions about it.

DR. S.: Tell me what happened in school today with Joey.

MAX: I was shooting him with my pencil.

DR. S.: Why didn't you stop when he told you to?

MAX: I kept shooting him because I thought it was funny.

DR. S.: Did Joey think it was funny?

MAX: I don't know.

DR. S.: Did you want him to laugh?

MAX: Yes.

DR. S.: So you did this to get him to laugh, but he wouldn't?

MAX: That's right. He was supposed to laugh but was just yelling at me.

DR. S.: So he should have laughed at you, but he didn't. So you continued, hoping that he would laugh. He didn't do what you wanted, did he?

MAX: No. He was being the boss and telling me to stop. I'm supposed to be the king.

DR. S.: Well, Max, I think there is a problem here. Number one, there are no kings in the U.S. It's illegal. However, we do have bosses. Parents can be bosses. Teachers can be bosses. But seven-year-olds are rarely bosses. [We discuss this in much more detail.]

MAX: But Joey was being a boss!

DR. S.: No. Joey was telling you not to annoy him. That's a right that we all have. You were breaking the rules. You are not allowed to bother someone like that.

MAX: My sister bothers me.

DR. S.: Well, that's another story. We'll talk about that one when we finish this one. Let's talk about what you are the boss of. You decide lots of things. For example, what shirt you are wearing. You picked out your own sneakers. [We discuss lots of other examples.] There are also things that you are not the boss of, like what time you go to bed, or if you'll go to school. [We discuss more of these.] So you see, there are some things you are the boss of and not others. Let's talk about Joey. You wanted him to laugh. That was your rule for him, and he wouldn't follow it.

MAX: That's right. He was supposed to follow my rule; my brain told me that.

DR. S.: Well, Max, that's another thing that you are the boss of, your brain. Let me show you. No matter what I tell you, you tell your brain to ignore me. Ready? Okay, Max, lift your leg. Hey, how come it didn't move?

MAX: (*Laughs*) I told it not to. [We do several more examples of this.]

DR. S.: That's right. And you can tell your brain to leave Joey alone and to follow the rules in school. You need to be okay with this idea. This really solves a problem for you. It doesn't make it worse. Do you understand what I mean?

MAX: You mean I can't be the boss.

DR. S.: That's right. Let's write this out on a card for you:

MAX CAN'T BE THE BOSS OF EVERYTHING.

MAX CAN ONLY BE THE BOSS OF HIMSELF, NOT OTHERS.

MAX CAN BE THE BOSS OF HIS BRAIN AND TELL IT WHAT TO DO.

MAX CAN USE HIS BRAIN TO SOLVE PROBLEMS.

Step 2: Expanding the Concept: Once some easy changes have occurred, and being okay has become an accepted concept, you begin to move up the ladder of difficulty to more problematic situations.

You may have to "push" some changes by saying, "You need to be okay about . . ." He needs to begin to "think" differently about the situation. He cannot tell himself negative things about the situation or why he can't do it. Instead, he needs to tell himself how it might be okay doing something different, and how it could turn out to be okay, just like the other things he has already tried that have already turned out okay.

In your discussion you establish a hierarchy of difficulties. You never start with the most difficult, always something small. You gradually move up his hierarchy of difficult situations. Don't stop after doing one situation. As you continue to use this technique, don't be surprised if your child tells you that he hates being okay. He may say this when you are asking him to do something that is particularly difficult. Let him know that he can call it by any name he wants (see step 3), but he still has to be able to deal with changes in his life. These positive changes you are asking for will be the cornerstones of how well his current and future life will be.

Step 3: Using Other Phrases: After you have introduced the concept of being okay, you can discuss it using a shorthand phrase that summarizes or captures the essence of "being okay." For example:

- *You can be okay.*
- *You need to be okay.*
- *It's okay to be okay.*
- *Can you be okay?*
- *Make yourself okay.*
- *Tell yourself what you need to be okay.*
- *Just do it and be okay.*

Use other phrases if they seem better suited to the specific situation, such as:

- *Just do it.*
- *Bite the bullet.*

- *Good choice versus bad choice.*
- *Switch gears.*
- *Be flexible.*

Step 4: Adding a Visual—A Self-Talk or Prompt Card: This concept can be used as a separate, free-standing technique or as part of this overall process.

You can give your child a written card to look at that summarizes a concept or contains the essence of the goal you want to achieve. For example, the card can say, I CAN BE OKAY, EVEN ABOUT SOMETHING I DON'T LIKE. I CAN SAY "OKAY," AND THEN BE OKAY, WITHOUT GETTING UPSET. Eventually this becomes the new thought process. For some, what is on the card is memorized very quickly and the card is no longer needed. Others may resist the notion of something being written down, and not even want to look at it. Some may want to throw the card away. In this case, not writing it down can be an enhancement to his doing it, i.e., being okay.

Sometimes a social story will need to be created to facilitate the change. This, a much longer version of the prompt card, is discussed in chapter 8.

Step 5: Using Props, Toys, Objects, and Activities: Some children will be particularly resistant to change, and you may have to use additional strategies. These children are often strongly oppositional and/or become highly agitated and upset with any attempts to change things for them. They need some transition steps to reach the final goal of being okay. They need an object, prop, toy, or activity that makes the change possible. This object or activity reduces the distress. To gain access to the object or activity of his desire, he must perform some action that you have set forth. The discussion sounds like this:

"You need to _____ [the necessary action] if you want _____ [the desired object or activity]. You will not get _____ [the desired object or activity] if you do not _____ [the necessary action]."

Access to the desired object or activity does not have to be all or none. It can be given or taken away in increments.

Step 6: Aiming for Successive Approximations: Achieving successive approximations allows for your child to do some part of the task, or another simpler task that "moves the child closer" to the task you want. For example, writing a response rather than saying it, or talking about something while standing rather than sitting. This is often needed for children who are highly resistant, rigid, and oppositional.

Step 7: Intervening in the Middle of a Crisis: Sometimes situations devolve quickly into your child throwing a tantrum. In this case you will need an incentive to enhance being okay. Without one, the likelihood for success decreases.

The incentive needs to be something he wants, enjoys, and craves with passion. It is often an object or activity that he has obsessed on. It should be something that is easily given and removed.

The crisis stage usually involves some form of upset or tantrum, marked by crying, anger, and the like. It is usually over something he desires or something that he wants to avoid. Tell your child that he needs to stop crying so that you can discuss with him how he can obtain his goal. Ignore the tantrum, and periodically repeat the same phrase: "When you are finished crying, we can *discuss* what you want." Eventually he will say he wants to talk. You repeat that he needs to stop crying before you can discuss it with him. When he has stopped, you will have him restore the environment (fix anything that was knocked over, etc.) if necessary, which further tests his compliance as well as determines if he is really okay. Tell him he needs to be okay, which means doing certain specific behaviors, which you spell out. They should be few in number and very concise. Tell him that he must complete those actions or you cannot discuss any concerns. Do not go too quickly down this road because many children act as if they are calm, but are not, especially when you once again begin to discuss the initial problem.

Step 8: Reaching the Continuation Phase: You will know where you are in this process by the degree of difficulty you have each time a new situation is confronted. Continue with new experiences for your child, getting him to be okay. Any issue can be included at this point. When this is done easily and willingly, the process can continue on its own, with less effort on your part—that is, fewer prompts, shorter discussions, and less resistance. The beginning stages are always the hardest, with the latter ones occurring with relative ease.

6

Generalization and Sabotage

HOW TO MAKE CHANGES THAT LAST

"Practice Makes Perfect."

For some parents, survival is all that matters. To get through the day without a major upset is often considered a successful day. But this is not sufficient. You and your child need to thrive, not just survive. Without the development of new skills that can be used every day, real growth will be limited. You want your child to repeatedly demonstrate appropriate skills, to apply them to new situations, and to function as productively as he can. To do these things, your child or teen must be able to use his new skills in a variety of settings with a variety of people.

Billy was an eleven-year-old who was quite rigid, especially when it came to doing anything new. Everything that he liked had to stay the same in his life. If he stopped once at McDonald's on the way to my office, he wanted to stop every time. As he was taught to be more flexible, he was able to accept changes in his routine. Christmas vacation, however, was a big problem. It seems that each year his family went to Cancún over Christmas. This year was to be different. They were going to Disney World due to extenuating circumstances that could not be altered. Billy was quite beside himself with this prospect looming in the near future.

His mother tried to placate him by telling him about all the wonderful things he would experience in Disney World, but to no avail. He complained, argued, cajoled, and threatened his parents with bodily harm if they did not change the plans back to Cancún. With several weeks yet to go before the trip, his anger was slowly building. Each time his mother told him of some other glorious event or ride in Disney World, his tantrum became worse.

In desperation, his mother finally informed me of the situation. Before Billy and I began our conversation about his pending trip, I first gathered the above information about the trip, observed a brief discussion between mother and child as they discussed the trip, and only then started to talk to Billy about this problem. By taking these steps, I found out details about the situation, such as what had already been discussed and what were future possibilities regarding vacations. We talked about his being stuck and his need to be flexible. Remember, this concept of flexibility had been discussed before and implemented for other situations, so it was not new to him. I needed for him to see that the current situation with Disney World was similar to past events about which he had needed to become more flexible.

I told him how this was another event where he was stuck and that he needed to understand it as being similar to many other events. Therefore, he needed to solve it the same way: get unstuck, be flexible, find another solution to his problem, and be okay. I became a sphere of influence—someone who was going to help him solve a problem and make it better. I pointed out how he was making this issue into a large problem; how large problems had often ended up badly for him in the past; how when he was stuck before he had become violent; and how being flexible, keeping it small, and getting unstuck makes things go better. Once I made the connection for him and he accepted my advice, his anger subsided and it became clearer to him how he was making the situation worse, how he needed to accept the idea of going somewhere else this year, and how Cancún might be a trip to take at another time (knowing that his family goes on frequent vacations). He calmed down and was able to go to Disney World and have a good time without any further upset.

This chapter will help you increase the effectiveness of the changes that you have made so far. In order for them be permanent, you need to work to:

- Have your child or teen use his newly acquired skill *more than just one time*.

- Have your child or teen use his new skill in *different situations* or with a *variety of people* other than you.

- Make sure that the new skill is not lost or forgotten over time.

Generalization and *sabotage* are two techniques that will help you achieve these three goals. Both of these assume that your child has already begun to demonstrate his newfound skills. He must be able to use a skill in a specific situation more than one time before you teach him how to generalize the skill to other situations.

Generalizing a skill is not the same as learning the skill in the first place. These are two distinct tasks for you to work on. You cannot teach generalization until a skill has been initially learned. This initial learning process may consist of a number of repetitions of the new skill in exactly the same situations. When your child seems to have grasped the idea of what to do in that first situation, you can begin to show him how to generalize it to other situations. If you do not teach him how to generalize he will not be able to do it. Your child sees each event that occurs as separate and unrelated to every other event that he has ever encountered. He does not comprehend how two situations could be related or how he can use a skill he has previously learned in another situation. You must draw the parallels between events, point out similarities, and "connect all the dots."

We all know that just because a skill has been learned and used once or twice, there is no guarantee it will continue to be a tool used by your child. To keep the skill "alive" for your child, you must use sabotage. This is the act of intentionally creating situations in which your child demonstrates the skill in increasingly more difficult scenarios that you have created. Let's look at these ideas in more detail.

Generalization

As noted above, once a skill is learned in one situation, it tends to be used in another only when one recognizes the similarity between the two situations. If the *content* of the events is different, people tend not to see the events as related in any way. This will be especially true for the Asperger child or teen. What he learned in one situation will have no bearing for him in the next situation. This makes it difficult for him to use new skills across settings, as well as to learn from his mistakes. You will need to help your child see that two situations are related and that the same skill can be used again. Remember that events or situations can be similar because their content is the same, such as doing homework on Monday night and doing it again on Tuesday night. However, two events can also be the same because their *underlying issues* are the same, even if their content is different. It is especially important for you to help your child see this connection.

For example, an underlying issue can be *doing what someone asks you to do, dealing with surprises,* or *being flexible.* So, in our situation, let's imagine that Bob learns how to be okay and not throw a tantrum when something unexpected happens, such as his plans change with regard to going to the movies. In a second situation, his plans change about where he will go for dinner. To the Asperger child or teen, these are not related events. One involves the movies and the other involves a place to eat. You will need to show him that both situations involve a *change in plans* (the underlying issue) and that he can respond in the same way to both of them. You can say, "When plans change, Bob, and we are going to do something different than what we had originally agreed to, we have to be flexible and not get upset. You know how to do this because you did it with the movies, and going to dinner is similar. You need to handle it the same way." Again, you are reinforcing that the content was different, but the underlying issue of making a change was the same. You help him by:

- *Pointing out the similarities between two situations based on their content.* For example, each dinnertime or every time he sits down to do homework, he will do the same thing or act the same way; or, how the same response is needed for two different settings because of their underlying similarities.

• *Using phrases that have been applied before as a label to a new skill.* For example, telling your child, he needs to "be flexible" about this situation, just like he was in the other situation or at that other time. When you developed a new skill with him earlier, you explained why it was needed, how to do it, and what not to do. All of these ideas are now wrapped up in the label that you use to describe the skill: "Just do it," "Be okay," "Don't get stuck," or whatever. You may use any of these phrases, or you can invent your own. Just make sure you use them consistently so your child can learn how to generalize.

It is easy to become confused and not realize that the underlying issue is very important. You may miss this idea because you are focusing on the content only. Generalization can only occur when you and your child realize how different events, with the same underlying issues, require the same strategies and skills to resolve any difficulties. These underlying issues are the reasons for the behavioral difficulties you see and will be the ideas you will focus on to develop generalization. Remember that an Asperger individual's behavior is usually a function of the difficulty he has with moving on and letting go of an issue and thereby "getting stuck" on it. His anxiety about this situation leads to his rigidity and it is the most common reason for his behavioral problems and manifests itself in numerous ways. Once we are clear on this issue, we are ready to teach generalization.

How to Generalize a Skill

In previous chapters we discussed teaching a new skill to your child or teen. When you were working on a new skill, you learned it was important to label the new skill, using key phrases as prompts and cues. For example, when you were trying to have your child do a better job with homework, with less arguing and procrastination, you talked with him about doing things differently. You mentioned how often his behavior started an argument with you, with lots of yelling and threats. Instead of the assignment taking forty-five minutes, it took two hours. So you proposed another method to him to solve this problem. Instead of arguing and delaying the completion of the homework, you spelled out for him, perhaps in writing or with a social story, that if he cooperated and got it done in forty-five minutes, he'd have more time to spend on a preferred activity, like using the computer or reading. The usual way of doing homework could be called a "bad choice" and the new way could be called a "good choice." Or, you could say that he usually does better in dealing with a problem when he is "not stuck" and is "flexible." Your entire discussion with him is captured in the phrases that you have used to label the new skill. It does not matter what the label is. It only matters that you use this phrase the next time a problem occurs. When it is time to do homework once again, tell him *before* the event that you want him to make a "good choice" or "not get stuck" or be "flexible." This will remind him of what he did the last time and how to do it again.

Once he has mastered this skill for this task, you will use this technique for other events unrelated to homework, where he has to make a "good choice" or where he needs to be "flexible." If necessary, you may have to explain again all the parts that make up the phrase you are using. This is okay to do. You can do it this way as many times as you think are necessary. Don't be surprised if at some point your child says that he knows all of this already. Just remind him that he must show you, not just know it in his head. Soon, he will begin to use these new skills in other situations, as long as you are reminding him *before* the situations by using the appropriate phrase. Each time a situation occurs that is similar in content or in the underlying issue, you will prompt your child with the phrase he has learned and he will be able to use it effectively. You will have taught him a new and appropriate behavior to replace the old and inappropriate one. Remember that you must practice every new skill a number of times for your child to learn it. Don't expect him to learn a skill and demonstrate it after one discussion. It needs to be practiced many times over a relatively small time span—days and weeks. As time goes on, he will need less prompting from you to remember what he has to do, and will begin to do it without reminders. As the reminders and prompts decrease, he will be learning how to generalize the new skill. It will be more fully generalized when he demonstrates it without any prompting or he points out the problem in others as well.

Sabotage

Once your child has begun to generalize his new skills and use them in a variety of settings and your day-to-day life has calmed down, you can begin the next phase. Remember, the next phase, called *sabotage,* is never done when things are still in turmoil. Most of your child's life must be stable without very many tantrums, disruptions, upsets, or arguments. Only at this time can you begin to consider using sabotage.

The difference between learning a new skill, generalization, and sabotage is that the first two are usually worked on with naturally occurring events. These are the normal events of your child's life that occur without you doing anything to make them happen. With sabotage, you intentionally create problems for your child to solve. You do this so your child can practice and reinforce his skills. If you do not reinforce these skills frequently, they will gradually disappear. You must constantly, gently push your child forward, and this is done through sabotage.

Each time you begin to target a behavior with sabotage, you start small and slowly move up your child's hierarchy of difficulty. This is a list of events or situations that have caused upset for your child in the past. For example, if your child experiences anxiety in dealing with other people, ordering his own food in a fast-food restaurant is generally easier for him to do than returning an item to customer service in a store. In the first situation, it is pretty obvious what needs to be done. Returning an item to customer service has variables and nuances that make it less predictable and therefore produces more anxiety. As you move up the list, if a problem occurs, you review what was successfully done before and then try the task again. If successful, you begin to move forward again up the hierarchy. Never increase the level of difficulty if you experience problems. Sabotage should always be built on prior successes.

Planning for Sabotage

CSIT emphasizes the importance of *planned* sabotage. Your child will now make use of all the prevention techniques that were previously introduced. For these new skills to become a part of your child's daily repertoire, change must be orchestrated, and you must set the stage for this to occur. By doing so, you are able to control your child's exposure to change, as well as the application of these new skills. Obviously change cannot always be planned (indeed, this is the core reason life is so difficult for those with Asperger's syndrome); dealing with times of unplanned change will be discussed in chapter 8, "Crisis Intervention." However, our belief is that practicing planned change will increase your child's ability to generalize his skills during times of unplanned change. By doing so, he becomes more flexible in both his thinking and his actions.

As you introduce planned change/sabotage, your child may become more anxious. This can be manifested in one or several of the following ways:

- Crying, verbal or physical resistance, tantrums, aggression

- An increase in rule-bound behaviors or increased insistence on routines and rituals

- An increase in obsessive-compulsive behaviors

- An increase in self-stimulatory or tic behaviors

- An increase in persistent behaviors or restricted interests (often seen in language use or centering around an already established area of special interest)

- An increase in perfectionism and in inattention/distractibility/impulsivity issues

When beginning sabotage you need to make sure that your child's increased anxiety does not interfere with your efforts. You need to maintain structure in those parts of your child's environment not affected by the planned change. Change only one thing at a time. When he has had success with one change, additional changes can be introduced. When initially selecting an issue to sabotage, select a small event that occurs frequently. Some children may be ready to attempt multiple changes on a daily basis, while others may only be able to successfully accept changes on a monthly basis. Either way, planned change should be introduced on a daily basis. With some children it will be a minor change (trying a bite of a new food); for others it will be a major change (playing with a group of children at a playground). With some children it will be the same change introduced over a number of days; for others, it will be many different changes introduced over a number of days. The important variable is that planned change is introduced on a regular basis and rewarded.

If other events will be occurring during your attempt, wait until your lives have calmed down a bit. You may never get complete tranquillity, but some stability is important. Examples of major changes might include: home changes (parent away, new sibling, moving, holiday or vacation time, guests visiting), school changes (new school, new teachers, new or increased mainstreaming), and physical changes (new medication, illness). Don't attempt sabotage during times like these.

When you are introducing the planned change, use concrete language, as well as verbal and visual prompts—hand signals, cue cards, cue phrases, schedules, social stories, pictures, language scripts, posted rules that provide a "road map" for the activity, a posted step-by-step outline for task completion, and so on. In other words, develop a plan with your child, outlining how the sabotage will be accomplished. Resistant behavior will be significantly reduced if he agrees to the sabotage plan prior to it actually occurring. It is always a good idea to discuss issues with your child before undertaking them. People often want to just plunge right in without very much preparation, and that's never a good idea.

Remember Adam from chapter 4, who would only play with his beloved Lego sets if all the pieces were available? After using the strategies discussed in that chapter (flexibility, hierarchy of change) with Adam, he was ready for us to begin planned changes. The first step was to remove one or two pieces from one of his Lego sets without his knowledge prior to his playing with that set. Once he was comfortable with this, we increased the challenge level by doing it again, but this time when he was going to play with the Legos with another child. In this manner, we continued to gradually increase the challenge by removing more and more pieces from different sets and doing so when he was involved with different children. Each step helped Adam to internalize this skill, so that real generalization could take place.

It is important that your child understands and can complete all the steps involved in the task or activity. Make sure that nothing is beyond his ability and he knows how to do what you will be asking him to do. If something is too hard or hasn't been mastered, you must back up and reteach all needed skills in a step-by-step fashion prior to the introduction of sabotage. You may need to reintroduce guided practice, modeling, role-playing, and rehearsal.

If anxiety is increasing, your child may begin to engage in increased nonsense talk. Interrupt it, label it as inappropriate, and model more appropriate language. This should also be done if tone or volume become inappropriate. If a tantrum occurs, this must be worked through before the planned change can continue. Never move faster than your child as you attempt to teach skills. However, once the tantrum is resolved, the task or activity must continue. Tantrums cannot be seen as a means to avoid change.

You need to realize that sabotage may be difficult, but do not back down or give up. Remain calm, caring, and consistent. If planned change is introduced or addressed by a person different from whomever did the initial teaching of skills, this individual must be aware of how the skills were taught and use the same language.

If possible, allow your child to have some choice involving the planned change. This helps him regain a feeling of control. However, only offer this choice if it does not compromise the change you are fostering. Be immediately aware of any increases in your child's anxiety level in order to be able to intervene with previously taught anxiety-reducing interventions (being okay, keeping problems small, problems and solutions, social story). Your child needs to know and believe you are there to help him with completing the change, but not with avoiding the change. The message you want to give him is: *Change is happening, you will need to adapt, and I have given you ways to do that. I am here to help you, not cause you more upset.*

When introducing a planned change, have it occur *prior* to a familiar activity that your child enjoys doing. Thus, the completion of the change (a nonpreferred activity) becomes the motivator that leads to the enjoyable activity (a preferred activity). If his obsession or special interest can be incorporated into the sabotage activity (either as part of the activity or as the rule for the activity), he will be more likely to complete the initial activity. In fact, the change or nonpreferred activity might become a preferred one.

Age is not a factor when introducing changes. Introduce the idea of flexibility and change even to young children. Make sure it is in a concrete and visual manner, with flexibility seen as a desired goal. For children, storybooks or films that address this issue are perfect; for the older child or teen, a social story would be appropriate. When sabotage is successful, then link it to flexibility. To behave in a flexible manner becomes a rule. As Adam said in chapter 4, "I'm flexible, I just don't like change."

Flexibility through Sabotage

Once you have begun the change process and controlled anxiety that could destroy your efforts, you are ready to teach flexibility. You want your child to reduce his rigidity and do things differently and, of course, more appropriately.

Remember to begin with small issues. Try to control where and when your child can engage in particular routines, interests, and rituals.

Simultaneously, provide alternative behaviors. For example, if your child has a particular object he likes to carry, the rule might be, "You can hold your plug when you are in your bedroom. You can hold it for twenty minutes a day. You can decide if it will be twenty minutes at a time or if you want to break up the time." Or, if he needs to name all the titles of books a particular author has written you can say, "People don't want to hear all the book titles by [that author]. When you are talking about one of these books, the rule is, you can name two other titles, but only two." If you can't be successful with small issues, you are not ready to deal with larger ones.

You can introduce the idea of flexibility by presenting it in terms of a social story or being okay. For example, you would say, "Sometimes we drive to the mall and eat at McDonald's and sometimes we drive to the mall and eat at Burger King. This is a change and this is good. If I always pick the same restaurant I am being a 'me first' person. [Recall "me first" from page 79 in the list of key words and phrases we have found to be effective.] I need to be flexible about where we eat."

If your child has special fears, you will need to gradually desensitize your child to them. This was discussed above in terms of moving up your child's hierarchy of issues from smaller to bigger. For example, if your child has a fear of dogs you would initially write a story or make a chart (again, some type of visual, depending on which technique has previously worked with your child) outlining how you do and do not behave around dogs. You would also introduce some pictures and stories showing positive interactions between dogs and children. You would then role-play with your child, showing him how he is going to act with a dog, using a stuffed animal as a prop. After reviewing the written material and role-playing successfully, a real (well behaved) dog would be introduced with the adult present to provide necessary prompting.

Again, these sessions would take place with less and less adult prompting before exposing your child to dogs at random. Overcoming fears is another important aspect of flexibility. Remember, it is anxiety and fears that cause rigidity, and flexibility is the new behavior we want your child to learn.

The Asperger child or teen usually has special interests that are unusual and dominate his time, and this can be another area to address with regard to flexibility. It is important to help him be flexible about engaging in these activities. With activities that are socially appropriate, we have less need to eliminate them from his repertoire and more of a desire to have him be flexible about his degree of involvement. We don't want him spending all of his time doing them, however. If the activity is not socially or age appropriate, we would want even greater flexibility on his part in reducing their occurrence. Some activities that are more socially appropriate include playing computer games, rule-governed board games, and card games; completing mazes; collecting; Scouting; making models; and playing with Sega, Nintendo, and Game Boy and construction toys like Legos, Constructs, and Playmobil. It is very important to introduce other games and activities that involve gross motor skills, especially ball skills and sports. This is necessary for "blending in," both at and outside of school.

You can also introduce flexibility by teaching him "shades of gray," mentioned earlier. Sometimes we have an immediate need for him to be flexible, and we may ask him to do something right away without any discussion—"Just do it." This phrase becomes your child's cue for immediate compliance with no questions asked. As with other strategies and phrases, this must be practiced with your child and he must agree to it. All those involved with him must be aware of this phrase and know when to use it. Initially, it may be necessary to write the phrase on an index card and post it. You will know generalization has been achieved when your child begins to ask, "Is this a 'just do it?'"

Being flexible can be used for any transitions or resistance-to-change issues that your child is having. In this way, you are transforming an issue that your child sees as negative, enabling him to look at it in a new, different, and more positive way. You are providing a plan.

Remember, when you have achieved stabilization and you have begun to successfully sabotage events and situations, you will need to increase the degree of difficulty if you want to see the most growth in your child's ability to be flexible. The sequence of steps to take when you are going to do this is as follows:

1. Make sure things are stable before you begin to "mess things up." Be certain that the number of tantrums is small and the degree of upset is minimal.

2. Prepare your child for the change, deviation, and mix-up in a typical event by saying that something different is going to happen, but don't say what it is. In this way, he knows something is coming tomorrow, but he is not sure what it is. Then, when this new thing occurs, you let him know that this was the situation you were talking about.

3. Increase the intensity of the change by making it a real surprise, something that isn't ongoing or typical. It's a new or rarely occurring event. But, again, he isn't prepared for it.

4. The greatest degree of difficulty will be the disappointment. First, it can be a prepared disappointment, as in step 2, and then a surprise disappointment, as in step 3. This will be an event that is eagerly anticipated but does not come about.

In all of these steps, never move to the next one until you are satisfied that the one you are working on has been mastered. It may take reviewing of previously learned skills, but it should always be done slowly and carefully.

Once you and your child have developed a good working knowledge of the skills in the foregoing chapters, you will be ready to deal with the most difficult topic, covered in the next chapter, "Developing Social Skills." All the skills learned to this point will need to be utilized in the social arena.

7

Developing Social Skills

MAKING AND KEEPING FRIENDS

"Nothing's Easy."

On a pleasant Saturday morning in July, I am awaiting the arrival of six five-year-olds with Asperger's syndrome, members of my newly formed social skills group. Developing social skills is the most difficult area for these children, and the summer months, which often lack structure, are especially difficult. Because of this, I feel the weight of their parents' expectations. Even with all my years of experience, I worry. Can I mold these children into a cohesive group? Will significant behavior issues arise that may interfere with the group's activities? Will my "ocean" theme engage the children? Will the parents be able to help their child practice their newly acquired social skills at home so that generalization can occur? Despite my concerns, I'm excited about starting a new group.

The children begin to arrive and events proceed smoothly for a first session. The novelty of new people, a new environment, and new materials cause an initial increase in anxiety for the children, which results in an increase in problem behaviors. For example, one child doesn't want to leave his mother and throws a tantrum because this group isn't part of his Saturday morning plan. Another child refuses to sit in the second chair because he is always number four. After addressing these issues, we eventually settle in our beach chairs and I present our daily schedule (this is all visual, as discussed in chapter 4).

I describe the purpose of the group to the children, saying, "We are going to learn how to make friends and how to be a friend. Kids have fun playing with other kids, but sometimes it is hard to know how to play with them or what to do."

A very verbal, bright, and logical boy named Ethan immediately replies, "I hate kids. I don't play with kids. I only play with grown-ups. I'm not a kid. I don't like kids. I was born a grown-up."

My quick response: "Well, that's why you are here, Ethan."

Of course, changing someone's behavior, in essence their thinking, will not be that easy, and Ethan spends most of the first session making his position about other kids clear. It is obvious that Ethan's vision of himself as a grown-up and his belief that he hates other children stem from the anxiety he feels when interacting with other children. He has discovered that the adults in his world make him feel much less anxious. Why? Because the adults are willing to let him control his interactions with them, and they are more tolerant of his behavior than his peers are. If I can't change Ethan's thinking, my activities on how to make friends will never be accepted by him. Moreover, if he does agree to interact with other children without changing, his statements will not win friends.

I already know from the brief time I have spent with Ethan that he is a "logic boy," which means my approach must be logic based. My first goal is to help Ethan accept and verbalize that he is a kid. What can I use to appeal to his logic? My first thought: a dictionary! After our session I find a definition that I can use to help him change his thinking—now I have my prevention strategy.

The next Saturday morning I eagerly await Ethan's arrival. When the children first arrive, they engage in free play under the direction of my coteacher. I use this time to take Ethan aside.

"Hi, Ethan, I'm happy to see you. I want to show you something I brought." I hold up my dictionary with a smile. "Do you know what this is?"

Ethan quickly replies, "The dictionary, I love dictionaries. They tell you exactly what all the words mean and it can't be wrong." (Ethan has just reinforced my belief about the importance of rules and logic to the Asperger individual.)

I reply, "That's right, Ethan, but I read something in here that confused me, so I want to read it to you. But first, I want to ask you something. Are you all finished growing or do you think you will be getting any bigger?" (By initially acting confused and asking questions, we can learn how someone views a situation, and this understanding helps us to plan our strategy.)

"Oh, no, I'm going to get much bigger. Did you see my dad? I'm going to be as big as my dad before I'm done," Ethan replies, holding up his hand to illustrate his point.

"Well, Ethan, that must be why I'm confused. I looked up the definition of an adult" (I turn to the definition and begin to read) "and it said, 'a person grown to full size and strength.' But you just said you're still growing, which is what I thought. I'm worried. If you keep telling people you're an adult, they are going to think you are all finished growing and will not be getting any bigger." A look of worry spreads over his face and I can see the wheels in his head turning. I continue, "You do know that children grow into adults. So, if you tell people you are a kid or a child, you are also telling them that you are still growing, but when you finish you will be an adult." (I have purposely added the word *kid* to the discussion, because it gives him the choice of using a word other than *child*.)

Ethan takes a moment, then says, "Guess what, Mrs. Grayson? I'm a kid, because when I say that, people know I will become an adult. That's a rule."

"You're right, Ethan." And I smile, knowing I have started to move Ethan down a long winding road. He has accepted an opportunity to be flexible and allowed the introduction of change into his thinking. Now I must continue to move him along this road. The real work must follow, as he begins to learn how to socially interact with other children, without the burden of constant anxiety.

Remember, theory of mind (knowing what the other person will likely say or do) and perspective-taking combine to give a person *social intelligence,* which equals the individual's social thinking, understanding, and expression. Because the Asperger child or teen has difficulty in all of these areas, we understand why they find social situations especially anxiety provoking. Anxiety reduction can be accomplished by direct instruction, coupled with many opportunities to generalize these new skills in real-life social situations.

In addition, because social skills change with age, the instruction will need to be ongoing. Just like other skill development areas, this will be an area of continuous development as your child learns to maneuver in the social world. Your child will be unable to "go with the flow," will lack an awareness of social cues, will have great difficulty engaging in reciprocal social interactions, will be unable to use or understand most nonverbal forms of communication, and may also lack the desire to interact with others. Furthermore, though your child or teen may fall into the Asperger subgroup of those with a real desire to interact, they often engage in inappropriate social interactions because of the skill deficits mentioned. The "hidden agenda," or social thinking behind social situations, must also be taught.

It will be impossible to develop social skills without also developing *social thinking* and *pragmatic language* skills. Social thinking refers to the behaviors and rules we use in our social interactions (how a winner should act after a game, how to initiate a conversation). The verbal and nonverbal communication we employ in social interactions is called pragmatic language (in addition to the words we use, this also includes voice tone, facial expression, and body language). These two areas must work together for a child to have successful social interactions. We quickly process what is going on around us, then immediately formulate and execute a response. Most children learn these skills through observation and by interacting with others—very little of it is taught. Unfortunately, this is the most problematic area for the Asperger child or teen. Without direct instruction paired with generalization strategies, learning will not occur. Therefore, it is important for your child to receive direct social skills training, paired with techniques to foster generalization in all social situations he or she will encounter. This can and should take place anywhere and anytime: at home, at school, or in a therapeutic social skills group. However, certain guidelines must be followed and specific strategies used to achieve effective social skills training. Let's explore what a good, comprehensive social skills program should look like.

Developing Social Skills

General Guidelines

To date there is no one program to teach social skills. While more and more programs and materials have become available, you will most likely have to pull from and modify several to meet the needs of your child. In addition, because social skills requirements constantly change due to situations and people, teaching will have to make use of "teachable moments"—in other words, seizing upon each and every opportunity to teach social skills whenever real-life circumstances present themselves.

DEVELOP PLAY SKILLS FIRST

When you begin working with your child on social skills at home, you will teach him using a one-on-one (child/adult) model. If your child is young, you need to determine if he has "play skills" before you can begin teaching social skills. He should be able to play alone using varied objects, such as blocks, cars, and action figures. Is he able to be flexible and use his imagination during play? Be very observant. What may look like imaginative play on the surface may actually be the replaying of a previously viewed TV program or video or a rigid verbal script your child has developed that he continually replays without change. You will need to teach and practice imaginative play with him prior to beginning social interactions with his peers. Besides knowing how to interact with a peer, your child must also know what to do with the objects being used. Is your child able to use the toys in the way they were made to be used, as opposed to, say, lining them up or otherwise incorporating them into a ritual?

INTRODUCE PLAYMATES

Once these have been worked on you should introduce one other child. Be creative: if peers are not available, think about another member of your child's class, a cousin, a sibling, or a neighbor's child. But it is critical that you select the right child for these initial interactions. A child who is too passive may allow your child to control the interactions, and a child who is too active may overwhelm your child. Have him practice turn-taking skills when involved with peers. This would involve various toys for younger children and board games for older children and teens. Be aware of your child's special items, usually toys, games, or objects related to his special interest areas. It may be too difficult for him to share these items and, therefore, these should be removed prior to a friend coming to visit.

If your child is part of a larger group, the members of the group should be *as close in age as possible,* no greater than a span of two years. It is important to remember that the social skills needed at age five will be quite different at age eight. Furthermore, the techniques outlined (starting on page 158) demand a certain level of intellectual functioning and language processing. The techniques will be most effective for those children and teens who fit the diagnostic criteria for Asperger's syndrome (average or above IQ levels and no significant general delay in language). The skills we are presenting are specific to this group, and an Asperger child will rarely benefit from techniques designed for the autistic, attention-deficit, or emotionally disturbed child.

DEVELOP SOCIAL SKILLS OUTSIDE THE HOME

It is important that you extend your structured, one-on-one training with your child to include interactions with peers outside of the home, in a variety of social settings. Using structured lessons and following a social skills curriculum will never be enough by themselves to make these skills permanent.

At a minimum, you will be working on this with your child weekly. However, it is very important that the techniques you have taught during your direct instruction be reinforced throughout each day by everyone else who is involved with your child. Without this, there is no guarantee that your child will ever learn to generalize these skills. This is another example of how important it is to communicate with everyone involved with your child: relatives, teachers, caregivers, siblings, and so on. Social skills training can only be as good as those providing it. To be effective with social skills training, all the people principally involved with the child must:

- Have an understanding of Asperger's syndrome

- Be a good observer of both the child with Asperger's syndrome and his typical peers

- Be aware of the role that anxiety plays in the area of social skills

- Be aware of the effect that secondary behaviors (obsessive-compulsive behaviors, rigidity, self-stimulation, etc.) have on social skills development

- Be able to teach these skills directly and in the moment

COMBINE SOCIAL SKILLS TRAINING WITH SCHOOL

If your child is in school, a social skills group should be part of his educational experience there. The school is the ideal place to provide direct social skills instruction for multiple reasons: it is the social setting that will be the center of most of your child's social life, peers are readily available, and there are many daily opportunities for practice and generalization. Whether or not the school is the direct provider of your child's social skills training, his teacher should be well informed of the training so that she will be able to help your child with generalization of his social skills. If you want him to generalize in real-life situations, you must plan to directly teach this step on a daily basis.

The importance of "blending in" with peers cannot be overlooked. By "blending in," we mean not just acting, but looking age appropriate. The Asperger child or teen does not respond to—is not even aware of—peer pressure. He won't stop wearing a shirt with Thomas the Tank on it simply because peers are no longer wearing these shirts. He won't stop watching a Winnie-the-Pooh video just because he is now in sixth grade and this is not what other kids his age do. He won't notice that other students do not bring umbrellas to school. He will not notice that his classmates are listening to a particular singer or that everyone is talking about a particular movie or TV show. This is one of the areas where you must act as a "defender of reality" for him to make sure he is fitting in with peers in terms of clothing, accessories, and the latest craze: what's "in" in books, toys, games, videos, TV, music, and so forth. The idea is not to inhibit your child's individuality, but to make sure he isn't an easy mark for teasing because of his disability. As one father said, "I don't want to send my son to school every day with a target on his forehead."

General Techniques

The techniques described here should be an integral part of any social skills program for those with Asperger's syndrome. Use them when applying the core curriculum of social skills training that begins on page 165. Every such program needs to include the following:

- Using visuals
- Role-playing

FIVE GENERAL GUIDELINES FOR SOCIAL SKILLS DEVELOPMENT

1. Those teaching social skills must be thoroughly familiar with Asperger's syndrome.

2. Training must be tailored for each child.

3. Social skills training must be taught directly.

4. Teachable moments—those natural opportunities that unexpectedly occur (such as trouble coping with losing a board game or abrupt changes in schedule or routine)—must be utilized to develop generalization.

5. Training must be ongoing and evolving to adapt to your child as he matures.

- Supervised practice in real-life situations

- Generalization of skills

- Scheduling and arranging play dates or leisure activities

- Keeping current

- Learning to use peers as role models

- Addressing behavioral issues

USING VISUALS

For the young child, each new skill must be introduced with a visual. As discussed in chapter 4, you can use pictures, photographs, key words and phrases (such as those listed on pages 77–80), storybooks, social stories, cartoons, videos, and others to initially present a skill. The visuals should show both the correct and incorrect way to display the skill. If practical, these visuals should remain displayed, to be used as a prompt and/or as a visual reminder. This will not be as effective with adolescents, with whom the use of explanatory conversations (with cue cards or a social story) becomes more important. Using a popular TV show, movie, or video that depicts an actual social situation where your adolescent is having difficulty can be highly effective; however, it can be quite time-consuming to find the appropriate clips. Some commercially available social skills programs have developed checklists and forms geared to the adolescent.

ROLE-PLAYING

Next the skill is role-played both correctly and incorrectly by the adult. While role-playing, you are also providing the "language script" to be used in the social situation. Initially scripts should be specific and very explicit: tell the child exactly what he is to say and do. It is important to gear role-playing to your child's age. During your initial role-playing exercises, you may have to be quite dramatic and actually exaggerate your behaviors. Remember, it is often difficult for the Asperger child or teen to see subtle behaviors. The first time my speech therapist and I demonstrate eye contact, we have a conversation and never once look at each other. Most of the children, when asked what we are doing wrong, fail to notice the lack of eye contact. Instead they may say, "You did not have a nice tone of voice," or "You were not talking about something Mrs. Grayson was interested in," or "You were talking too much." They rarely notice the lack of eye contact until it is pointed out or quite exaggerated. You could easily model this activity at the dinner table.

Now your child is ready to role-play the skill, using the previously presented language script. First, your child would role-play with the adult. If this is successful, he would then be ready to role-play with a peer. During these initial role-playing exercises, prompting from the adult is often needed. This prompting would take the form of either holding or pointing to a previously used visual or using one of the previously used key words or phrases. However, this prompting will need to be quite subtle as your child grows older. With the older child, we often suggest a prearranged cue or code. The skill would not be considered mastered until the child could do it with a peer without any adult prompting. We will often videotape this step, especially if the child is having difficulty.

SUPERVISED PRACTICE IN REAL-LIFE SITUATIONS

The most important step would be giving your child opportunities to practice and use the skill in real-life situations. You will have to observe the interactions carefully to make sure the child is successfully using the skill. You will need to be close enough to actually hear what is being said. An interaction may "look" good, but when you actually hear what is being said you may find the interaction is not appropriate. (Again, the older the child, the more subtle you will need to be in your observing.) We often find that no matter how well the child can use the skill in the instructional setting, he has great difficulty transferring the skill to a real-life social situation because of his anxiety. You may need to prompt or reteach the skill. This must be addressed before the next social encounter.

GENERALIZATION OF SKILLS

Remember, "playing with a friend," "making a friend," and "being with a friend" are overwhelming skills for the Asperger child. Even after these skills have been taught, he will not understand how they translate into, "I want you to go to the mall with Tim," or "Today when we go to the playground I want you to play with the other children." This final step is the most abstract and, even after direct instruction of specific skills, will need to be taught in a step-by-step manner. Initial social interactions, whether at home or school, should have a dress rehearsal. Also, early attempts should only involve your child and one other peer. It will take time and practice before they are ready to be part of a larger group of peers. (Unstructured outside play with a group in the neighborhood will be the greatest challenge for a young child. Going to the mall or a party will be the greatest challenge for a teen.)

Role-play what the activity will look like: What will you say when your friend first arrives? How will you suggest activity choices? How will you decide what you will do first? What if you can't agree on what to do? What can you talk about with your friend? (You must practice these conversations and often provide actual scripts.)

For these initial interactions, rule-governed games or structured activities work best. With young children make sure these initial interactions are short and minimize the adults involved. (You are more likely to monitor the situation more carefully if you are not busy entertaining the other child's parent. However, if you are the only adult present make certain you are free from other distractions that could interfere with your monitoring of the interaction. You will be amazed by how quickly an interaction can go badly!) With teens, initial interactions should also be short, but most likely adult involvement will not be appropriate. Remember to take your cues from the parents of your child's peers. If they are allowing their teen to view a particular TV show or movie or play a particular computer game, though you may not like it, you should consider the possibility that this activity may be appropriate for your Asperger teen. This would extend to music choices, clothes preferences, concert choices, curfew times, as well as which activities are chaperoned and to what extent. As mentioned, learning how to make and keep friends must become part of the daily routine. It becomes a rule or task, just like getting dressed or completing homework. Some Asperger's children or teens will have little or no interest in social interactions. If this is the case with your child you may find it useful to use other activities or rewards as reinforcers for social interactions. (After you go to the birthday party you can have extra computer time.)

SCHEDULING AND ARRANGING PLAY DATES OR LEISURE ACTIVITIES
Once you are ready to schedule play dates (for young children) or social interactions (for teens) for your child, try to arrange them on a regular basis. Weekly would be ideal. In fact, we feel this kind of interaction is a better use of time for the Asperger child than homework or most therapies. Remember, Asperger children like routine, so making this play a part of the routine should help to increase compliance and decrease behavioral issues.

Arranging play dates if your child is young will be relatively easy and under your control. This will not be true once your child reaches adolescence. If he already has a network of peers this will be less difficult. If not, the best way to initially develop peer relationships would be involvement in a club or organization. (This could be at school, through your community, or through a temple or church.)

KEEPING CURRENT
If your child is young, fill your home with the latest and most interesting toys and games. This will make other children more likely to accept an invitation and return again. (The first child to have the newest hot video game among my son's friends always had a full house.) With teens make sure the activities planned are age appropriate and be available to provide transportation. Teens watch and discuss shows like the ones on MTV, though you may not like or approve of it as a parent. The difference between your teen and the typical teen is that they may be hiding this and other activities from their parents and yours is not. This is partially due to the increased involvement you have with your child by

circumstance and partially due to the honesty the Asperger individual displays.

LEARNING TO USE PEERS AS ROLE MODELS

Once your child is interacting with peers, help him to use them as role models. The older the child, the more able he will be at doing this. We find social monitoring is especially useful when in public. We provide the following rule: "When you are out with your friends, watch them. If you are doing something and no one else is doing it, then stop doing it." Try to be as specific as possible. For instance, if your child tends to laugh inappropriately, this becomes one of his social rules: "If your friends tell a joke or see something funny, make sure you stop laughing when they do." If they are going to a sporting event, say, "Remember to watch your friend at the baseball game. If he stands and cheers, you should too, but when he stops and sits down, you should too." Again, present these as "rules."

ADDRESSING BEHAVIORAL ISSUES

Be aware that behavioral issues will be present in every novel situation. Issues of rigidity, control, and obsessive-compulsive behaviors will reappear during social interactions and must be addressed. If not addressed, these behaviors will interfere with every attempt to facilitate social interactions.

Keeping these guidelines in mind, let's take a look at how these guidelines are applied in two different scenarios.

Scenario 1: You have arranged a "play date" for your child and you are ready to do some specific planning for this event. You will need to role-play with your child what this will "look like." Develop a schedule for the visit, come up with a list of possible play choices, develop some language scripts, and decide if certain special toys, the computer, or areas of your house will be "off limits." However, flexibility will have to be introduced into all these ideas, as another child is involved. You will have to discuss with your child the possibility that the schedule may need to be changed and he will have to "be okay" with this. Discuss and role-play what "being okay" looks like. You should also come up with a plan if they are unable to decide on a play choice, on who will go first, or who will use particular toys or game pieces. Your child will need strategies to solve these types of potential problems. All these events must be discussed and role-played prior to the visit.

Scenario 2: Your teen is ready to play a pickup game of basketball (after much individualized practice) with some other boys in the neighborhood. However, he would rather play computer games alone after arriving home from school each day. You present this new activity in the following manner: "You have lots of jobs in life. At school, some of your jobs are to follow teacher directions and observe the school rules. At home, some of your jobs are to put your clothes in the hamper and take out the trash. Another job you have at home will be making friends with some of the other boys in the neighborhood. I know you really like to use the computer after school, so I don't expect you to do this every day. I do expect you to do this one day a week for a half hour to start. Which day of the week would you like to select?" (Here you are giving your teen a choice and therefore some control.)

When he selects the day, you begin to write this information down. You are providing a visual and the needed "road map." "Okay, you selected Thursday. When you arrive home from school on Thursday, you will put on shorts and sneakers and go to Ted's driveway. Did you notice that is always where the boys play? What will you say to the other boys when you get there?" (Review, if necessary.) "Tell me what you do in a game of pickup basketball." (Review, if necessary.) "What will you do if the boys say you can't join the game?" (Review, if necessary. It will be very important that he has strategies to use when problems arise.) Remember, your child must be able to role-play each step with you, if he is to be successful with his peers. Of course, it will be very important for you to have some skills in this area. Practice these skills away from his peers until they are improved. If he can't improve his skills in this area, you may have to choose something else to do for peer involvement.

The Core Curriculum

This core curriculum is arranged developmentally, but two important reminders are in order. First, many of the goals are ongoing and will be worked on over and over again. The only change is the way in which the goal is addressed, which will change as your child matures. Second, you will be adding your own goals to this list to meet your child's special needs or as issues arise in the social situations in which he is involved. The core curriculum presented here can be easily copied and integrated into your child's social skills goals for school.

1. WHAT IS GOOD COMMUNICATION?

- **Eye contact—thinking with your eyes.** You are teaching that your eyes let your partner know who or what you are thinking about and eye contact lets others know you are interested and/or listening. You do not just teach "look at me," but rather why you need to make eye contact and what information it provides.

- **Personal space—thinking with your body.** You are teaching the correct distance from another when sitting, standing, and walking. Again, you do not just teach personal space, but rather, what information your body can provide.

- **Voice volume—thinking with your voice.** You are teaching the various voice volumes that can be used and where each can be used appropriately.

- **Tone of voice—"the way."** You are teaching that "the way" we say something greatly affects the meaning. You demonstrate the various tones that can be used and where each can be used appropriately.

- **Turn taking—think about me/think about you.** You are teaching that conversations are reciprocal and must consistently go back and forth.

- **Body posture—thinking with your body.** You are teaching correct body posturing when speaking to another person, when getting the attention of another, and when joining in with another. You teach that your body and the body of the person you are engaged with provide information to help you better understand the interaction and allow you to communicate more successfully. You are teaching the understanding of body language.

2. CONVERSATIONS

- **Introductions.** You are teaching how to introduce yourself, as well as friends and family, to others.

- **Conversational skills.** You are teaching that conversations have three parts—initiating, maintaining, and ending a conversation; that you start a conversation by getting the other person's attention; that conversations are about interests people have in common; that certain topics are not appropriate conversational topics; that you must stay on the topic of conversation; that conversations go back and forth (they are reciprocal); that you must both ask questions and make comments during a conversation; that in conversations you often "say what you see"(talk about an event, item, person as you see it happen); and that conversations must have a clear close or ending point.

- **Conversational rules and scripts.** Due to the complexity of this area you will want to develop some generic conversational rules, which your child can use as a guideline. These will include: say the person's name before you begin talking to them as a way to get their attention, look at the person you are talking to, face the person you are talking to, listen to what the other person is saying, and do not begin to speak until the other person has finished speaking. You can also develop generic conversational scripts, again that your child can use as a guideline. This could include questions you might ask a friend when you see them on the weekend, such as: What did you do this week? When did you do that? Who was with you? Where did you go this week? Your goal is to give your child ideas to start and then to keep a conversation going. It will also be important to teach the current idiom or fad sayings.

● **Different types of conversations.** In this advanced skill, you are teaching social conversations (ones that chiefly involve "small talk") versus formal conversations (ones that have a direct purpose).

3. JOINING IN AND PARTICIPATING WITH A GROUP

● **Asking to play with others or asking others to play with you.** You are teaching the language script and the actions that will accompany your words.

● **Responding when others don't want you to join in.** You are teaching the language script and the actions that will accompany your words.

● **Responding to teasing.** You are teaching the language script and the actions that will accompany your words.

4. INTERPRETING AND REACTING TO FACIAL EXPRESSIONS AND BODY LANGUAGE CUES

● **Identifying various facial expressions.**

● **Identifying various body language cues.**

● **Understanding what various facial expressions and body language cues tell us.** This is much more important than the identification. You are teaching empathy. How do they feel? How do you know that? What could you say or do in response?

● **Monitoring your own facial expressions.** You are teaching that your facial expression must match the situation at hand. Do you laugh when others laugh? Do you show concern when others are upset?

5. "GOOD SPORT" SKILLS, GAME PLAYING, AND GIVING AND RECEIVING COMPLIMENTS

● **How to be a good winner and loser.**

● **Game-playing rules.** There are multiple steps in this area, besides the ones specific to a particular game or activity. Consult the example of "How to Play a Game" included in chapter 4 and appendix C as a generic model.

- **The language to use in game playing.** You are teaching language scripts. How do you suggest game ideas? How do you begin to play? How do you maintain the play? How do you end the play?

- **How to handle conflicts and disappointments during game playing.** You are teaching problem-solving skills. Disappointments and conflicts might include: not being first or the particular number you want to be, not getting the piece or character you want, not playing the game you want, not following a preconceived idea you have for the way the game or activity will go, not following a preconceived language script.

OTHER SPECIFIC INTERACTION SKILLS

- **Asking for help.** You are teaching awareness of when this is necessary and the language script to be used.

- **Offering to help.** You are teaching awareness of when this is necessary and the language script to be used.

- **Sharing.**

- **How to interrupt appropriately.**

- **How to apologize appropriately.**

- **How to complain or disagree appropriately.**

- **Telephone skills.**

IMPORTANT ABSTRACT SKILLS

- **Understanding abstract language.** This includes idioms, metaphors, jokes, sarcasm, and similes.

- **Understanding another's point of view; making an impression by what we say, what we do, and how we act.**

- **How to solve problems and make decisions.**

- How to engage in conflict resolution and cope with anger.

- How to respect differences.

- How to resist peer pressure.

Special Tips

While, as we mentioned, there are a number of good commercial programs available, there is no one program that will meet all your needs. Rather, you should choose from various programs. Included in Appendix H are some commercial programs we have found to be especially helpful. Below are some materials we have also used.

Social Stories: For all of the skills mentioned above, social stories, which you develop together with your child or teen, can be a useful way to initially introduce each skill or to clarify a particular situation for your child. In general, social stories are useful both as a prevention strategy and when introducing new skills. We will discuss these further in the next chapter.

Eye Contact: When working on eye contact with young children, use "eye finger puppets" (available in most speech/language therapy catalogs). Play a game, having the eye finger puppets look at various items around the room. Point out to your child that you can tell what a person is thinking about by watching where that person's eyes are looking, and that when your child is talking to another person, he or she needs to be thinking about that person.

Personal Space: When working on personal space with younger children, we have found that placing a hula hoop on the floor, and then having two children stand on the inside with the backs of their feet against the hoop creates the perfect conversational distance. We also use "conversational feet," a pair of feet patterns taped to the floor, to designate the correct place to stand and how to orient your body to another when having a conversation.

Voice Volume: When working on voice volume, create a visual wheel that has a dial or arrow attached. Use this as a prompt to tell your child which volume he should be using. With the older child, rather than a wheel, use a scale from 1 to 10. Relate this scale to the volume control on a TV, DVD, CD player, video player, computer, or radio.

Turn Taking: When working on conversational turn taking with a younger child, pass a ball or microphone back and forth. The person holding the object is the speaker and when they finish speaking they immediately pass the object to their partner. This provides not just a visual prompt, but a tactile one as well.

Conversation Parts: When working on the three parts of a conversation with a younger child, we use the images of a traffic light to represent the three parts. Green light starts a conversation, yellow light maintains the conversation, and red light ends the conversation.

Topics: When working on appropriate topics for conversation we use a topic jar or bowl (a fishbowl used for this purpose always generates interest), and we have the child generate the topics to be put in the jar or bowl. Usually, the child will want his special interests to be included, and this creates a natural opportunity to discuss what are and are not appropriate topics of conversation. The rule is: only those topics placed in the jar or bowl can be used in conversations with peers.

Using "Wh-" Questions: When working on conversational skills, using "wh-" questions (who, what, when, where, why, and how) is useful as a way to foster questions and comments. Initially these should be written on index cards or a poster board.

Strategies

Let's look at a few examples that illustrate how to teach social skills. In each of the examples below, you should notice how each skill is presented in the same step-by-step manner. Each starts with a visual. This is followed by the adult modeling and role-playing the appropriate and inappropriate responses. Next, the child, with prompts from the adult, role-plays the situation. The adult and child continue to do this until the child no longer needs to be prompted. At this point, the child is ready to use his newly acquired skills in real-life situations.

SHARING

1. First, provide visual examples of sharing. Show your child pictures of children sharing and also pictures of children not sharing; have your child appropriately label the pictures. Reading a storybook about sharing would serve to enhance comprehension of this concept.

2. Now role-play for your child examples of sharing and not sharing. While doing this, also provide the language script (the words) to use when sharing.

3. Next, have your child role-play appropriate sharing with you. She should be using the language you presented previously. When she is able to do this without any prompting from you, set up a real situation that will allow her to do this with a peer. Continue to provide these experiences until your child is sharing without difficulty or prompts. If difficulties persist, continue to provide ongoing practice in multiple settings. Carefully observe your child to determine which particular aspect of sharing is difficult for her. Once you have this information you can begin to plan additional skill development.

PERSONAL SPACE—THINKING WITH YOUR BODY

1. First, describe this concept, again using pictures to show examples of appropriate and inappropriate use of personal space. The use of storybooks with younger children can be quite effective. Remember, in your discussion it will be important to include the reason for using appropriate personal space.

2. Next, model physical examples of appropriate and inappropriate personal space for your child. As mentioned, use a hula hoop or

"conversational feet" on the floor (masking tape works well, too) as a visual prompt that can be paired with the verbal prompt: "thinking with your body."

3. Now your child is ready to demonstrate the physical model. Initially, use the visual or verbal prompts, but fade their use as quickly as possible.

4. Once your child can successfully use the skill with you, provide real-life opportunities for her to use the skill with her peers. Again, you may need to initially prompt, but work toward fading prompts in order to achieve mastery of this skill.

INITIATION OF PLAY WITH A PEER

This is an example of what will be one of the most difficult skills for your child to develop. "Making a friend" or "playing with a friend" is especially overwhelming for the Asperger child. Although you may have taught all the individual skills, he will not understand how these skills translate to "Today I want you to find a friend to play with when we go to the park." This final and abstract step will need to be very specific.

1. First, playing with friends must become part of your child's daily routine, part of his daily schedule.

2. Your introduction of this skill to your child would be presented in this way: "At home you have many jobs. You dress yourself. You put your clothes in the laundry basket. You do your homework. Well, another job is to make friends and learn how to play with them. I know this is hard for you, so let's start with one day each week for you to work on this job. Which day do you want to pick?" Here you are giving your child a choice and therefore some control. At this point, you begin to write the information down. You want to begin to make it visual. You can use a social story format, a chart format, a schedule format, or whatever you like. Based on your knowledge of your child, select the format that seems to work best for him.

3. "Okay, you picked Wednesday. On Wednesday, we will go to the park and you will walk up to a child there and ask him to play with you." (If your park does not have readily available play equipment, make sure your child brings some items with him.)

4. "Will you bring a basketball or your trading cards?" (Again, you are giving your child a choice, but you are controlling the choice. Also, you are making sure to select activities you know your child is able to successfully do and that are also currently popular with his peers.)

5. "Now, what will you say to get your friend's attention?" (Review any part of this skill that your child is unsure of.)

6. "Do you remember how to play basketball at the park with a friend?" (While you review the rules, remember to add situations that may occur outside of the basic rules, providing your child with strategies to handle these.)

7. "What will you do if the first person you ask to play basketball says no?" (It will be very important that your child has strategies to handle this response. He will need to know how to respond if the other child asks to play a different game or does not wish to play at all. Hopefully, you have already covered this in direct teaching and you are just reviewing or practicing immediately prior to your child using it. If this is your child's first exposure to being told "no," you will need to spend more time on it.)

8. As you progress through each of these steps, your child must verbally agree to each step. If he is not able to do this, you will need to stay at that step and work on gaining agreement. If your child cannot agree to this process at home with you, he is certainly not ready to try it with a peer.

Social skills development is and will remain the most challenging area for you and your child. This is true for a number of reasons: first, the development will need to be ongoing as your child matures; second, these interactions are abstract and ever changing, so new skills will always be needed. Furthermore, it may be difficult to find professionals in your area who can teach these skills. Many professionals who may be good with children are not experts in Asperger's syndrome or social skills training. This is partly due to the fact that so much of this training relies on the ability to make careful observations, the ability to look behind behaviors, and the ability to "teach in the moment." So not only do you have to make sure your child gets appropriate instruction and generalization, but you may also be the only person who knows what is appropriate. But the rewards are remarkable. We have seen many children respond to social skills training, and actually look forward to social interactions, make and maintain friendships, and successfully blend into the mainstream without support. In the end, their lives have been made richer and fuller.

However, no matter how hard you work to prepare for problem situations, you can't prepare for everything that might happen. What do you do when the inevitable meltdown occurs? How do you get through the crisis and, even more important, what do you do afterward? Chapter 8, next, focuses on crisis intervention. Here you will learn how to turn such occasions into an opportunity for your child to learn more appropriate ways to respond in the future.

8

Crisis Intervention

WHAT TO DO DURING A CRISIS

Regardless of the amount of prevention and skill training provided to your child, not all crisis situations can be prevented. A crisis could result from new situations, too many changes at one time, changes in routine without warning, missed or misinterpreted social cues, and/or failure to use coping strategies. This will lead to your child or teen becoming anxious. Tantrums and noncompliance will often be the result of this anxiety, caused by the collapse of predictability in his environment. CSIT's crisis intervention techniques help your child work through the crisis and teach him more appropriate responses in the future.

Let's look at a crisis situation from beginning to end to illustrate how you integrate these two goals. Furthermore, in this particular example, you will see how important it is to understand the reasons behind the behavior, as discussed in chapter 2.

Tyler, a six-year-old in my class, was an Asperger child who desperately wanted to have friends, but had no skills to achieve this. Each day was torture for him, as his repeated attempts to interact with his peers were rejected. My class had an opening and I used this opportunity to teach Tyler social skills in a very controlled and predictable manner. When a potential student was coming for an intake evaluation, I would assign Tyler as his "buddy." Prior to the visit (remember the importance of prevention), I would review with Tyler what the visit would look like and what his role would be with his "buddy." These visits went very well and the prevention strategies used gave Tyler a chance to practice and generalize the skills he had previously learned through direct instruction. I was even able to use some sabotage.

Eventually, one of these potential students, Ian, was selected to join our class on a permanent basis and I knew, based on his previous interaction with Ian, that Tyler would be able to act as his "special friend" for the first few weeks. This would provide comfort to the new student and give Tyler a greater opportunity to practice and generalize his social skills. But when I told Tyler that he could be Ian's special friend, he had a complete meltdown, even before I finished explaining the situation. He began to cry, then scream, and proceeded to tell me how much he hated Ian. His negative comments about Ian went on and on. Remember, his last interaction with Ian had been very positive. Obviously, I had missed something and we were now in crisis mode.

I had two goals. First, to assist Tyler in calming down, and second, to discover the reason for his meltdown so that we could work on more appropriate responses in the future. Because Tyler was quite loud and distraught we separated from the rest of the class. Again, because prevention is so important, my assistant and I have a plan ready for those times when a student needs immediate assistance. If a crisis happens, I can immediately intervene with the student while she can continue working with the class. This is something you must work out in advance, at both home and school and in both regular and mainstream settings. You may be thinking, "I don't have time for this. I have other things to do." My response would be, "This is going to happen whether you have time or not. Can you really accomplish your other tasks if your child or student is acting out?"

Once separated, I worked toward calming Tyler. I avoided touching him or discussing the problem at hand. In a very calm and even voice (a bit lower than my typical speaking voice), I said, "You have a problem and I want to help you solve it. When you are calm, I will help you solve your problem." That's all I said. I was especially careful to not respond to the many negative statements Tyler was making, for instance, "I hate Ian. Ian's stupid. Ian wants to kill me. Ian will destroy our class. Ian is an alien. Mrs. Grayson is stupid. Mrs. Grayson is a witch. I want to hit you. My mother hates me."

Instead, I calmly repeated my statement, and would continue to do so for as long as it would take for Tyler to calm down. When he finally did and began to respond to my statement, I asked him to complete one simple request to show me he was ready to work with me: to pick up a chair he had knocked over. This would show me he was ready to work with me. (These tasks, which I call "compliance tasks," can be almost anything. They are simple requests that, if completed by the child, let you know he has moved on and is ready to work with you. You could ask him to get a tissue to blow his nose, to walk to get a drink, or to bring you a pencil to write with.) He completed this compliance task without complaint and placed the chair appropriately. This signaled he was ready to work with me. Sometimes, I may use two or three requests, if the child tends to have many tantrums and has difficulty with compliance.

If he had continued to complain or cry or if he had picked up the chair inappropriately I would have known he was still not ready to work with me. I would have gone back to the previous stage and again attempted a compliance task when he appeared ready. However, he complied, so now we were ready for the second goal, discovering the reason for the behavior and teaching more appropriate responses for the future. It is important to remember as you move into step two and begin to work on the problem, your child may again lose control. If this happens, you must back up and go through the previous stages again.

Because this transition from step one to step two is fragile, it is important to give your child or teen some sense of control. (Remember, meltdowns are almost always due to anxiety, and anxiety usually increases when the child feels he has lost control.) You should allow your child to make some simple choices: "Do you want to work on your problem at the table or on the floor? Should we use the computer or just write it? Do you want to use white paper or blue paper?"

At this point, Tyler and I began to investigate his problem through discussion. Since I had not seen any environmental triggers I looked for internal ones and, based on Asperger subtypes, I knew Tyler was a "fantasy boy." As I explored this path, I discovered the reason. Because there were seven students in my class, Tyler had made our classroom into Snow White and the Seven Dwarfs. I was Snow White and each student was a dwarf. He had even assigned accurate names for each dwarf. Tyler was quite rigid and he could find no way to incorporate Ian into our classroom, because he would be the eighth dwarf, and there were only seven in the story. It had nothing to do with liking Ian or wanting Ian as a friend, which he did.

I had a few choices. I could pacify Tyler by selecting another student to be Ian's special friend. This choice, however, did not allow for any teaching or growth for Tyler. I could forbid him to discuss or have his fantasy, but I could never verify this, because I could not go inside his head. Finally, I could use this as an opportunity to work on Tyler's rigidity by increasing his flexibility. I would help him accept the possibility that you could have eight dwarfs. This choice, which is what I did, allowed Tyler to become more flexible, maintain an internal fantasy I could not control, and accept Ian into our classroom. He was also able to continue to work on his social skills, the most important goal. The reward was watching Tyler become a friend to Ian and having him whisper to me, "Guess what, Mrs. Grayson? Eight dwarfs are better than seven!"

Crisis Intervention Strategies

Certain steps must be followed when implementing any crisis intervention technique. The sidebar on page 179 contains the "Ten Commandments of Crisis Intervention." Examine these carefully. You must have a clear understanding of these guidelines. Your ability to follow these will determine your success or failure in crisis intervention.

While you can use various intervention techniques in response to a crisis, your reaction must remain consistent. Let's explore some specific techniques.

Problems and Solutions

Problems and solutions is a technique best used when your child is just beginning to display problematic behaviors, but is also quite useful as

THE TEN COMMANDMENTS OF CRISIS INTERVENTION

1. Have a calm voice and demeanor, but convey firmness.

2. Make it clear to the child that you are in control; don't plead or make second requests.

3. Help the child to see you as a problem solver. Let him know that you are aware of how difficult the situation is for him. Tell him your job is to help with this difficulty. Explain clearly that your help does not mean avoiding the situation or doing it for the child, but rather helping him to do it. E.g., "You have a problem and I am here to help you solve it."

4. Stay on topic during the crisis. The child may bring up extraneous or unrelated issues to try to justify his behavior.

5. Ignore or interrupt irrelevant comments. Respond with: "That doesn't make sense, I can't pay attention to that," or "That is off the topic, so I will have to ignore what you are saying," or "I can't help you with your problem while you are talking nonsense."

6. *Say what you mean and mean what you say* at all times during the crisis.

7. Keep your goal in mind as you go through the crisis intervention steps: creating new rules for responding in the future.

8. A step isn't completed until the child has given you his verbal consent to the conditions of the step. Be prepared to repeat steps if additional meltdowns occur before moving on to the next step.

9. Allow the child, whenever possible, to make choices as you move through the crisis intervention steps; however, do not offer choices if they would compromise what you are trying to achieve.

10. Practice/rehearse what has been decided as the appropriate solution to the problem; this may involve completing an activity or sabotage, accepting a change, or restoring the environment after a meltdown.

a strategy once the tantrum has subsided and the child is calm. The following steps describe how to implement this procedure:

1. Choose a private place to intervene.

2. Calm the child.

3. Label the crisis as a problem.

4. Provide choices.

5. Solve the problem.

CHOOSE A PRIVATE PLACE TO INTERVENE

It is important to select a private place to intervene. It will be more conducive to problem solving and will help your child "save face." This is especially true if the problem arises during the school day, on a playground, when peers are present, or in public settings. It becomes imperative if your child is having a full-scale tantrum. If a space is not available, try to separate yourself and your child as much as possible from others (e.g., find a corner, have your backs to other people). During this initial stage of the intervention, when your child is most upset, you must remain calm and focused on the task at hand. Your child or teen must know you are in control.

CALM THE CHILD

Do not begin the problems and solutions process until your child is calm. While the meltdown is in progress, speak using a minimum of clear, concrete phrases as I did with Tyler. Ideally, make use of previously taught phrases. Selecting one that can be repeated over and over is most effective: "I can't talk to someone crying. Get your control and then we can solve your problem," or "As soon as you have control, we can work on your problem." Do not allow your child to engage you in any off-topic or nonsensical conversations. Be prepared for this stage to last anywhere from five to thirty minutes. If this is the first time you have done this intervention with your child or teen, expect it to take longer.

As you use this intervention more frequently, you will be able to move through the steps quicker.

LABEL THE CRISIS AS A PROBLEM

While calming the child you began to describe his crisis as a problem. Once your child is calm (he stops crying, stops nonsense talk, sits calmly, looks at you, begins to talk to you calmly, asks for your help), you can begin to assist him with solving his problem. It is important to again reinforce that his crisis is a problem to be solved and that you are the problem solver: "You have a problem and I'm going to help you solve your problem." As discussed with Tyler, at this point you want your child to cooperatively complete at least one "compliance task" (e.g., blow his nose, pick up an item that was thrown, sit in a particular chair).

PROVIDE CHOICES

Because you want your child to join with you, attempt to provide some choices as soon as possible. This will help to refocus your child and begin to give him some sense of control. (Remember, noncompliance and meltdowns usually arise when the child or teen feels he has lost control and his anxiety increases.) These initial "choice questions" should center around solving the problem and might include selecting the color of the paper to be used to write out the problem, selecting the writing implement to be used, selecting the color of the writing implement—any minor choices that will move the process along without compromising what you want to accomplish. For instance: "Let's write your problem down to help us solve it. What color paper would you like to use— white, blue, or red? Do you want paper with lines? Should we use markers, a pen, or a pencil? Which color would you like?"

SOLVE THE PROBLEM

You begin by saying, "Now we are ready to talk about your problem, and how to solve it." Next, you describe in detail for your child what has occurred. At this point, you are using *cognitive restructuring*. You are reframing and reinterpreting the situation for your child. As you restructure the situation, you clearly outline both appropriate and inappropriate responses to the situation. Everything discussed is written down; the amount of words used will depend on the age and reading skills of your child or teen. With younger children or beginning readers, pictures would be important. A list or social story format is often effective. Below are two examples of how to use this technique.

The first example shows how a teacher would deal with a situation; however, you could just as easily apply this technique to one you encounter with your child. Let's imagine that your child has a favorite item he wants to hold while waiting for the bus at the end of the day. The rule is, "all items must be in your bookbag as you wait for the bus." As your child starts to pack up he leaves the toy out of his bookbag and the teacher hears him begin to verbally complain about not wanting to put the toy inside. The following steps would be followed.

First, she walks up to your child, gets on his level, and calmly but firmly says, "You have a problem and I'm going to help you solve your problem." His response will probably be to complain more about wanting to carry the toy. She ignores this complaining, does not yet touch the toy, and continues to say in the same tone, "You have a problem and I'm going to help you solve your problem." This may need to be repeated numerous times as your child's behavior continues to escalate. This small incident has now evolved into crisis state. This is not an unusual occurrence. As soon as the teacher sees any lessening of the child's inappropriate behaviors, she begins asking new questions to refocus your child and give him a sense of some control. ("Now we can work on your problem." "Where should we write?" "What color paper should we use?") This initial phase will last from five minutes or thirty minutes. Remember, if this is the first time she is using this technique with your child, it will probably take longer. These initial choice questions should center around solving the problem. Once your child is answering the teacher's questions, he can no longer complain and is beginning to focus on solving the problem.

Now she is ready to clearly outline your child's problem on paper: "You have a problem. You want to hold your action figure while you wait for the bus. The rule at school is that everything you are taking home is put into your bookbag before you leave the classroom. How can we solve this problem? Here are some choices: 1) you can put it in your bookbag now, but you can take it out when you are sitting on the bus; 2) you can leave it at home tomorrow and then you will have no problem; 3) you can talk to the teacher about the action figure while you wait for the bus; or 4) you can play 'I Spy' with some friends while you wait for the bus."

As she writes, she goes into more details regarding each solution based on her prior knowledge of the child. Once your child agrees to one of the solutions, the intervention is complete. If your child does not agree to any of the solutions, then an additional step is needed. She would say, "It is your choice to put the action figure inside your book-bag or not, but if you do not put it inside your bookbag then I will have to take the action figure and put it on my desk. That is what happens if you make a bad choice and then you will not have it tonight."

The key to this step working is the teacher's previous relationship with your child. If your child views her as a consistent, fair adult, he will be aware of the final outcome and select one of the good choices. If this is the teacher's first attempt with your child, she is planting the seeds for use in future interactions with him. If your child has a tantrum when she first tries, it is not a failure—it is the beginning of the learning process. We know this is difficult to go through, but staying with it will ultimately reduce the frequency and intensity of future meltdowns.

Our second example uses the technique to solve a problem "after the fact." Due to some circumstance that allowed your child to avoid the encounter, this did not escalate into a meltdown or crisis, but it could have. Although you could let this go without a discussion, talking about it can provide a good learning experience, and it can also precipitate a crisis as your child relives the event through the discussion. We suggest not to ignore the situation. Suppose you see your child playing outside in her neighborhood. A new child approaches her to play, a potential friend. The response of your child is inappropriate (say, your child spits at the child) because the new child's interaction has caused your child's anxiety to increase. Even though your child has been taught how to greet a friend, she was not prepared to generalize the skill in this novel situation.

Since this is "after the fact," your child is calm and you can immediately start to solve the problem. You would say, "You have a problem. You were riding your bike and another child in the neighborhood rode up to you and smiled. You made faces at the child, growled, and spit. This is not a way to make a friend. How can we solve this problem?" You begin to write up the problem, again giving the child choices in terms of the paper and writing implements to use. You continue, "You have a problem. You do not know what to do when new children come up to you when you are playing outside. The rule is to act friendly and give a greeting. To act friendly looks like: 1) a smile on your face; 2) looking at the child; and 3) saying to the child, 'Hello, my name is Jane. What's your name? I am [doing such-and-such]. Do you want to play with me?' You cannot growl, spit, or show a mean face. These are all bad choices and you can practice making good choices instead. This is being nice and making a friend." (Again, while you are writing, you would add more details regarding each solution based on your prior knowledge of your child.)

In solving these two children's problems, you may have noticed that there were four steps to the problem solving process:

1. Obtain verbal compliance.

2. Make sure the child understands.

3. Role-play and practice.

4. Reframe frustration, challenges, and changes as problems.

Crisis intervention is a series of sequential steps. Earlier steps may need to be repeated if your child is having difficulty with the later steps. It is important that you understand each of the steps involved in this process, so carefully read the descriptions below.

Obtain Verbal Compliance: At each step (reframing of the situation, developing appropriate responses, outlining inappropriate responses), having your child verbally comply is crucial. Do not proceed until your child or teen agrees with what is being written. He must do so verbally, and the more he is able to add to the discussion (describe what happened, give examples of appropriate and inappropriate responses), the more assured you can be that he agrees. If he does not agree to any of the solutions, additional steps need to be added. This could take the form of consequences that would be applied for continued noncompliance. For instance, "If you can't show me that you can be okay with being last sometimes, then you will have to be last all the time, until you can show me you are okay with being last." The key to this step working is how things have gone previously. If your child views you as a consistent, fair adult (in other words, a sphere of influence), he will be well aware of the final outcome and select one of the good choices offered. When there is a natural consequence that can or will occur if noncompliance continues, you need to point this out to your child so that he clearly understands that his situation will only cause more problems. Remember, if this is your first intervention of this kind, this step will take more time and may cause additional noncompliance and/or meltdowns. However, it is important to remember you are just not solving the crisis at hand, but also planting the seeds for future interventions of this type.

Make Sure the Child Understands: At this step, you must also check that your child understands what is being discussed. Make requests such as: "Tell me what I said," "Tell me what your problem was," "Tell me how you can solve your problem when this happens again," and "Tell me what you will do the next time you have this problem." If he appears unclear or expresses any confusion, this is the time to correct it.

Role-Play and Practice: Now that your child verbally agrees with and displays an understanding of what has been written, you are ready to role-play and practice/rehearse the new solutions that have been developed. Re-creating the situation that occurred or approximating it as closely as possible is important. You will need to go through this phase slowly and step by step. Often, the Asperger child is able to comply in the abstract, knowing that the real concerns (a ritual, obsession, routine) are not actually being compromised. Frequently, at this step, resistance will occur. You may have to go back to earlier steps to modify or add to what has already been written. Do not be afraid to revisit or repeat earlier steps, even the meltdown phase. If you do not take the time to do it now, you will guarantee a reoccurrence of the same crisis, without the benefit of any prior prevention or reframing of the problem. You would have lost the benefits from this intervention because you did not successfully see it through to completion.

Reframe Frustration, Challenges, and Changes as Problems: Throughout this intervention, you label frustrations, challenges, and changes as problems that you are there to help solve as the problem solver. In the future, when you see the child beginning to lose control, you start the intervention immediately and introduce the phrase "keep your problem small." You will say to your child, "Right now your problem is small. Let's start solving your small problem, before it becomes a big problem." Using your hands as a visual while speaking, to illustrate the size difference, can also be effective. Help your child remember how you worked together to solve his last problem. Remind him that the problem was not solved while he was upset, but was solved once he was able to calm down and use his words. You want your child to begin to realize that the "meltdown phase" is a time waster and the "solving-the-problem phase" is what will move the process along. Most Asperger individuals want life back to "normal" as quickly as possible and find these meltdowns as problematic as we do!

If you are consistent about using this technique, you will eventually see generalization initiated by your child when he begins to become upset by a situation. Your child will come to you saying, "I need a story [or list or some other device you've used]," or "I have a problem, can you help me solve it?" Finding what will work best with your child may require some experimentation and creativity on your part. We have already discussed using stories. A more visual technique to refocus your child is the problem wheel (see appendix D). The visual presentation of problem-solving questions on the wheel provides a way to move your child from frustration to problem solving. Even better, you will eventually hear, "I made a good choice and solved my problem," or "I kept my problem small."

Good Choice/Bad Choice

Good choice/bad choice is a technique that can be used as an alternative to problems and solutions. As mentioned previously, which technique you will select will depend on the subtype of the child or teen with Asperger's syndrome. Most factors discussed under "Problems and Solutions" continue to be needed here. The primary difference between the two techniques is one of language. The language used with good choice/bad choice is simpler, so this technique may be better suited for a younger child or those with more language/cognitive needs. The use of good choice/bad choice can also be easily incorporated into a social story, which is another technique we will discuss later in this chapter.

This intervention can be used before your child becomes significantly upset, when the first rumblings are heard or any mild dissatisfaction is expressed. Your careful observation and prior knowledge should allow you to recognize the first signs of a potential crisis. The phrases themselves ("good choice" versus "bad choice"), which you should have introduced previously during prevention techniques, serve as a cue to your child that he is beginning to lose control. You are letting him know you are there to help him; reminding him that he still has control, because he has choices to make. In addition, it is a time to remind him of the consequences of a "good choice" versus the consequences of a "bad choice." As with problems and solutions, you must remain calm and focused on the present issue. All extraneous conversation is ignored. You remain in control of the situation, while giving your child choices you select. These "choices" all have clear consequences. Your language is not only clear and concrete, but also as precise as possible. Here's an example of a "good choice/bad choice" intervention.

Peter, age ten, has been asked to leave the computer and proceed to a new activity. This request is immediately met with loud, verbal displeasure. If you were using good choice/bad choice, you would first move closer to Peter, get his attention, and say: "You need to leave the computer by the time I count to three. It is your choice to leave and move on to the next activity or not. If you leave, you are making a good choice and will be able to make other choices you like today." (Mention the reward system, if one is in place.) "If you do not leave, you are making a bad choice and will not be able to make other choices you like today." (Again, if possible, tie this to an established reward program.) The more consistent you have been with Peter and the more consistently you have used previous prevention strategies, the more effective this technique will be.

After this initial verbal exchange, calmly count to three. If Peter makes a good choice, immediately praise him for making a good choice and repeat that this means he will have other opportunities to make choices throughout the day. In addition, throughout the day whenever he has a choice or is engaging in a preferred activity, remind him of his earlier good choice. If Peter makes a bad choice, immediately respond with the consequence. Be prepared, because this might lead to even more resistance from Peter. You must be ready to add additional consequences or move on to problems and solutions in response to his behavior, which may become quite disruptive.

If having this conversation with an older child, it would sound like this: "Peter, your computer time is up and you need to move on to _____. It is your choice whether or not you leave the computer, but there are consequences if you don't leave now. Remember, this is what you agreed to. If you do not make an appropriate choice, then _____ will happen. Which choice are you going to make?" Again, as discussed above, your previous consistency with Peter will directly influence which choice he makes and how smoothly this is accomplished.

Social Stories

Social stories is a technique that was initially developed by Carol Gray. While there are now many variations available, I feel her original technique remains the cornerstone. This technique can be both preventive (used in anticipation of a situation you know will be difficult for your child) and crisis oriented (used as an intervention following a crisis, both to solve the problem at hand and to teach as a coping technique to be used in the future). Social stories provide the child or teen with a road map for what to do when encountering a new or challenging situation.

Social stories are never generic, but written with a particular child or teen in mind. They are specific to the child, in response to or in anticipation of a particular event. There is no such thing as "social story time," when topics are randomly selected and a social story is developed for a possible future need. (However, it is often beneficial to refer to the generic materials available if you are just beginning to learn how to write social stories. These generic samples will help to familiarize you with the format of a well-written social story. We highly recommend that you consult with the many excellent materials developed by Carol Gray (see appendix H).

If you're a teacher, eventually, when you have had repeated opportunities to successfully use social stories and feel comfortable developing them, a situation might arise that would lend itself to the development of a group social story that would benefit a whole class (in response to a specific playground problem, to enhance the following of a specific school rule, to clarify specific behaviors when in the mainstream).

General guidelines to follow when using social stories are included below. This is just a very brief introduction to the development and use of social stories, based on our own personal usage of this technique. The guidelines for using social stories are:

1. Develop the social story prior to the problem.

2. Allow the child or teen as many choices as possible.

3. Review the social story daily.

4. Consider using social stories for any situation.

Develop the Social Story Prior to the Problem: Ideally, the social story should be developed with your child or teen prior to the occurrence of the problem situation. When this cannot be anticipated and it is developed "after the fact," it must be when he is calm and can focus on the social story with you. Do not attempt to develop a social story until your child is calm and able to comply with at least one simple request (as outlined under "Problems and Solutions," earlier in this chapter). Remember to follow the rules of crisis intervention. Limit distractions and be prepared to remain with your child until the social story is complete. Sit next to him while working on the story.

As with any technique, remember that social stories will not be effective with everyone. When you initially develop a social story with a child or teen, you will be able to gauge the social story's effectiveness based on a few different variables. These will include: your child's interest in the social story's development, his verbal agreement to the ideas presented in the social story, and his compliance when the ideas in the social story must be implemented. This will quickly let you know if this is an effective strategy for your particular child. Readers, "rule" or "logic children," those who enjoy stories, those with stronger verbal skills, and those who like to figure out events and/or negotiate are usually the best candidates. Those who rip up the story are not!

Allow the Child or Teen as Many Choices as Possible: Providing your child with choices when creating a social story is critical, as long as these choices don't alter its intent. Most are quite simple: "Would you like to sit at your desk or at my table?" "Would you like to use paper with lines or blank paper?" "Would you like to use white paper or colored paper?" "What color pen would you like to use?" "Do you want to use a pencil or a marker to write the story?" "Would you like to type the story on the computer?" "Would you like to add pictures?" When the social story is complete, your child or teen is allowed to help make the extra copies that will be needed (this is often very reinforcing for the younger child). As you write the social story, allow him to select from choices you have offered; for example, "Instead of screaming when it is homework time, you could ask to use the computer or play a video game when your homework is completed appropriately. Which would you like to pick?"

Once again, when giving choices, always keep in mind the integrity of the social story you are developing. Giving choices involves more skill on your part and should probably be introduced after you have written a number of social stories and feel confident with social story development. To initially develop your social story writing skills, create the social story prior to the event and then review it with the child or teen before the event occurs. Once you feel comfortable doing this, you will be able to develop social stories with the child present or in response to a crisis situation. It would be helpful if you could find a mentor or colleague to review your initial social stories with.

Review the Social Story Daily: Once you have completed the story, read through the social story with your child at least once or twice. Then have him rehearse and role-play using the new responses developed in the social story. You may need to prompt or model for him during these initial rehearsals. Alternatively, after observing his response, you may decide you need to make revisions in the social story.

If the social story has been completed for a future planned event, it is imperative to review it on a daily basis, leading up to the actual event that the social story was developed for. This ongoing practice and reinforcement will be crucial to the social story's effectiveness and should be continued until the child's compliance is demonstrated without problems. Begin to read the social story less often only after his compliance becomes automatic.

Consider Using Social Stories for Any Situation: Remember, social stories can be used for any home, social, or academic problem your child or teen may encounter. If he has a special interest and you can incorporate that into the social story, it is certainly acceptable and will add to his interest in the social story. Phrases from Dr. Seuss, numbers, map symbols, and phrases from a particular foreign language are all examples.

If you're a teacher and the social story is a school-related issue, a copy of the story should always be put in the student's desk and additional copies should be given to all school personnel involved with the student (make sure you give a copy to the student's parents as well). If the social story involves a home issue, besides the copies made for the child and his parents, copies are always made for anyone else (teachers, therapists, relatives, friends, bus drivers) who may be involved with the child regarding this situation.

HOW TO WRITE A SOCIAL STORY

Having decided you want to use a social story, you now need to write one. How do you begin? Think of a social story as a story that describes a situation in terms of: the relevant social cues used and the behaviors needed in a particular situation; and a description of what the child or teen should do and should not do in a particular situation. The social story should be very clear and quite specific. Though reading ability is not required, due to the language involved, the child should be functioning above the moderately mentally retarded range of intellectual functioning. Here are the main steps to follow when developing a social story:

1. Target the specific situation for which you want to develop a social story. You will need to have as much information about the situation as possible and plan for variations that may occur (an event is canceled, someone gets sick). You must be familiar with the child so that you can understand their perception of the situation and what motivates them to respond in an inappropriate manner.

2. The social story should contain three basic types of sentences, and it may be helpful to practice writing examples of each type before you begin to develop your own social stories with a particular child. The three types of sentences include:

   a. *Descriptive*—These sentences clearly define where and when the situation occurs, who is involved, what they are doing, and why. It is important to carefully describe what people are doing and why they are doing it.

   b. *Perspective*—These sentences describe the reactions and feelings of others involved in the situation.

   c. *Directive*—These sentences describe the specific responses the child needs to make in the situation. Directive sentences clearly tell the child what is and what is not expected as a response to a given cue or situation. A directive sentence often begins with the words, "I can try to . . . ," "I will work on . . . ," and "I will try . . ." It is important to state directive sentences in positive terms—describe desired responses instead of simply describing problem behaviors. It will be necessary for you to model, rehearse, and role-play the desired behaviors. For instance, "Following directions looks like . . . " "Being okay looks like . . . " or "This is how you do your homework."

3. Remember to be aware of the child's age and functioning level as you create the social story. Use vocabulary, grammar, and print appropriate for the child's comprehension level. Don't be overly concerned with mechanics and proper use of English.

4. Write the social story in the first person present tense ("I go; I say") if possible, as though the child is describing events as they take place. It makes sense when writing a social story in anticipation of an upcoming difficult situation to use the future tense.

5. You may want to add illustrations, especially for nonreaders, but make the pictures simple, avoiding too much detail.

6. The Asperger child is often rigid and inflexible. Avoid using terms like *always*; instead use terms like *usually* or *sometimes*. When developing a social story, you have another opportunity to practice and use the concept of flexibility.

7. As you begin to develop a social story with a child, remember the power of a social story is directly related to your prior relationship (sphere of influence) with that child.

Always remember, the goal of a social story is not rote compliance, but to relieve anxiety by teaching social understanding and, thus, allowing the Asperger individual to use more appropriate responses in the future. Below is an example of a social story I used with a six-year-old boy who was afraid to go to the movies.

SAMPLE SOCIAL STORY
"Going to the Movies"

My name is Harry and I am a really great kid!! I do lots of things that kids do. I go to school, I play with friends, I go to the mall, and I play with lots of neat toys. One thing that kids like to do is go to the movies, that is really fun. You get to see a new movie as soon as it comes out and the picture is much better than when you watch it at home. You can also eat popcorn, candy, and have soda. After you see the movie you can talk to your friends about it. This is a great topic of conversation.

I used to be afraid to go to the movies, but I am not anymore. Being afraid of a movie does not make sense. When I go to my first movie, because it is my first time, I can hold Mom or Dad's hand if I feel worried. Also, because it is my first time, if the noise bothers me, I can cover my ears. I cannot talk or cry or ask to leave until the movie is over, that is the rule. I can pick where we sit and what I will have to eat and drink.

I will go with my family in November to see the new movie *Brother Bear*. This is not a choice. This is something kids do with their families. Because it is my first movie, if I do a good job, Mom and Dad will let me pick a special place to go after the movie. I think I will pick _____. Also, Mrs. Grayson will make me a very special traffic light sign.

I know I can see *Brother Bear* and make a good choice!!!

Planning for a Crisis

While reading this chapter is relatively easy, implementing the techniques, especially when in the middle of a crisis, can be quite difficult. Emotions are high and you just want to get through the crisis as quickly as possible and then quickly forget it. However, if you respond to a crisis in this manner, they will continue to increase because you did not address the reasons for it and teach your child alternative behaviors.

Try to remember the following five points when planning for a crisis situation with your child.

1. If you do not master the basic concepts, you will not survive the crisis. In other words, you will not be the one in control when a crisis occurs.

2. There are never great options during a crisis, but it does provide the child or teen with an opportunity to learn more appropriate responses. Often the Asperger individual learns quicker under these circumstances.

3. Remember there are two factors that will determine what happens during a crisis: your child's personality/subtype and your skills and personality. It is especially important during a crisis to match your intervention to your particular child's subtype. In addition, be very aware that if you have not yet become a "sphere of influence" in your child's life, these interventions will take much longer to successfully complete. Your child will continue to respond inappropriately and, based on prior learning, will respond to your new requests with an increase in the intensity and duration of his inappropriate responses. You will have to be quite firm and persistent when you initially begin to change the way you respond to your child in a crisis situation.

4. Please understand there is always a potential crisis out there somewhere. The most effective strategies are those that are well planned and ready to be implemented as soon as a crisis presents itself. Do not be fooled by "the calm before the storm."

5. If you use a crisis to teach your child more appropriate responses in the future, not only will your child be learning, but you will too. You will learn from the crisis and be better able to manage the next one, which will inevitably occur.

As a parent of a child with Asperger's syndrome, you probably agree that dealing with a crisis is one of your most difficult jobs. The next chapter will help strengthen your role as a parent. We will focus on parent empowerment, how to manage daily life more smoothly, and ways in which you can assist your child to successfully blend in with the world around him. The goal is to help you create a home environment that feels more stable and peaceful.

9

Reaching the Final Goal

"I'm Okay, You're Okay"

Your Role as a Parent

The number of people—children, teens, and adults—diagnosed with Asperger's syndrome has exploded over recent years and treatment approaches have moved from nonexistent to a myriad of philosophies. As a parent, you can and must become your child's advocate, supporter, and expert. There are many types of interventions, ideas, philosophies, and experts in the marketplace from which you can choose. It is possible to spend every waking moment consulting with another expert, getting a different opinion, planning a new course of treatment, or involving your child in multiple programs. It is also possible to be overwhelmed about what to do and end up doing nothing. You need to become a knowledgeable consumer, carefully evaluating and selecting how to help your child in the most effective manner. You need to talk to professionals and other parents, gather information, and become your own expert. You won't be able to do all of the above tasks by yourself. You will need to enlist professionals to help you.

However, it is not a wise idea to rely *solely* on the advice and direction of others. Through the process of learning about Asperger's, you alone will know in your heart who your child is, what his strengths and needs are, what works for him and what doesn't, and can create a step-by-step plan of how to help him.

You must constantly evaluate what the professionals are doing to see if your child is making any progress. It is very easy to spend years doing things that are ineffective. Use the following guidelines to help you determine if your child is progressing and improving:

1. Create a written description of the issues and concerns your child faces. Is he very rigid, too anxious? Does he argue too much or throw tantrums excessively? Use the questions Characteristics Checklist and Sohn Grayson Rating Scale in appendices A and B to help you complete your description.

2. Give a numeric rating to each of the concerns you have, indicating how much of a problem each one is. For each issue, using a 1–5 rating scale is often useful, with number 1 being a small problem and 5 being a big problem.

3. Date the information you have so you can look at these issues at a later date and compare them. You have now created a baseline measure of how your child is doing. As you begin an intervention, you will have a record of how he has been doing with regard to specific issues.

4. Determine the specific goals that the intervention is supposed to address. Do not accept treatment that has no goals, vague goals, goals you do not understand, or goals that have no functional relevance; that is, they do not impact on his daily life.

5. At varying intervals, perhaps every three months, you can rate your child again on those dimensions you're working on and compare them to your baseline data. You will give each issue your subjective rating using your 1–5 scale, or whatever way you measured them before, and see if any improvement is noted.

6. After two rating periods, six months, you will know whether any progress has occurred, no matter what your expert may tell you. If you do not see progress, discuss this with your professional and consider changing goals, treatment procedures, or the professional with whom you're dealing.

Keep Pushing

It is not unusual for parents and others to see progress and then become complacent. Never stop pushing ahead. Asperger children and teens will often experience relapses or stresses that cause them to temporarily lose skills. Constant practice of old skills and the development of new skills are needed.

If your child has not reached puberty, you need to realize that this life stage can exacerbate problems, and you need to prepare for it. If you have a teenager who is finishing school and will be going to college or getting a job, he will need to be taught how to be more independent. This skill is not developed overnight. Think about what you need to achieve with your child and teen and plan for it. It's often a good idea to start with your end goal in mind and work backward. For example, if you want your child to go to college, there is much more than grades involved for the individual with Asperger's. He has to become independent, be able to be away from home, be able to control his anxiety and obsessions, be able to problem solve, be able to handle his finances, know how to seek help, and so on. Each one of these tasks will require a step-by-step plan.

For example, being able to leave home can be difficult for many. Has your teen ever slept away from home or away from family members, and if so, for how long? If he has not, arrange for him to be away from home for gradually increasing periods of time. How has he done with the food that someone else served? If this is difficult, he needs to be in situations with others where he cannot dictate what he eats, and he has to learn to "make do" with what there is to be eaten. Has he been able to handle any problems that have arisen when he was away? He has to independently be able to handle surprises, disappointments, and changes without preparation from others. Did his anxiety remain at a low level? If not, he has to be able to self-calm. Did obsessions increase? If so, he has to learn to be more flexible. As you can see, every identified problem requires a plan to develop the necessary skills to overcome it.

Even if your child is years away from puberty or college, you will want to continue to work on skills. Each new day-to-day situation is a new challenge for your child. As your child progresses, hopefully the problems become smaller. Even though the issues become more subtle, he will still need your help. You will begin to use more of the generalization skills discussed earlier to help him see how many new events are just variations of old ones.

Balancing Other Demands

From the moment your child was identified with Asperger's, you have probably experienced the stresses of trying to do more things than you have time and energy for. This issue puts you in a dilemma: How much do you do and how much do you turn over to others? This is not an easy decision to make, but it is an important one. There is never going to be anyone else who cares as much for your child, knows him as well, or has as much at stake in his success as you. Teachers, therapists, case managers, psychologists, physicians, and others will come and go in his life. You are the constant. Learn as much as you can and use your knowledge to help him. Don't become overwhelmed by all that needs to be done. Take it one step at a time. It is inevitable that your Asperger child will take up more time than your other children, but don't leave them out. Time management and organization are important skills for parents, as well as their children, to learn.

Daily Life

As you learn what to do and how to do it, focus on the small picture as well as the big picture. The large picture is the goals you are working on, but these goals are made up of much smaller events and subgoals. Interventions are based on the multitude of small events that occur in your child or teen's life. These are the everyday events that can be easily ignored. Instead, begin to micromanage your child's life, especially until the teenage years. You will have much less opportunity to do this after your child becomes a teenager. Attend to the details of what occurs each and every day. There is no such thing as an issue or event that is too small. Everything counts. But don't think that you have to do all of them at once. Work on one or two goals at a time.

Medications and Other Supplements

Many individuals with Asperger's and their families will look to sources of help beyond therapies. They will look to medications, herbal treatments, vitamins and minerals, injections of various kinds, and diets. One form or another of these approaches will play a role in most Asperger individuals' lives, especially as the child becomes older. Something will always work for someone. However, you need to be extremely careful in selecting what you give your child. Many times, people base their decisions on word-of-mouth information, anecdotes on the Internet, or unsubstantiated information. We know how tempting it is to go with the latest idea, but it may turn out to be an ineffective fad or even be something harmful. Stick with proven results that have been scientifically tested.

It is not unusual for additional difficulties to arise as your child or teen matures. Depression is a common occurrence as your teenager realizes he is different from others and he becomes more isolated. By far, medications are the most common approach considered. In pursuing this avenue, you should realize that medication has positives and negatives. The negative aspects are the side effects they can cause, as well as their ability to exacerbate the issues for which they were prescribed. Sometimes medications cause more of the symptoms that you wanted to treat.

Many Asperger individuals are extremely sensitive to medication and they can easily be given too much. Always start at a very low dose and slowly increase the amount being given, looking for benefits and side effects.

When medication is given, it should be used to target specific issues. For example, if a child displays ADHD symptoms, he should receive medications that target those issues. On the other hand, a child who is rigid or obsessive will need a different medication. At times, he may need more than one medication. The task of matching the medication to the symptom is a complex job and best left to a physician who is very experienced in Asperger's and medications. However, when medication works, which it often does, it can cause a wonderful improvement in your child or teen.

What Is Success?

It is never enough just to get by and survive day-to-day. You want the individual with Asperger's syndrome to have feelings of control and competence in his environment; to be more in line with society's rules; to be less rigid, which reduces anxiety; to expand his narrow repertoire of interests; to have learned how to cooperate and accept others' rules; and to act with ever-increasing independence to be the best he can be. In essence, you want him to be okay.

At the same time, those working with Asperger children need to feel that everything is not a battle anymore. They, too, need to be okay. This is not to say that your child or teen is cured. Rather, everyone's life becomes better. Your child goes to school or work and returns home without many incidents. Surprises, disappointments, and changes are handled with relative ease. Social relationships are continuously improving. And life becomes a more cooperative adventure for all.

Perhaps the best way to define success is with one final example from one of our previous children. Jack was twelve years old and had considerable anxiety. He had virtually no interactions with peers. Most communication with others was brief and generally about topics of interest to him only. After some time of working with him, we decided medication was needed and he began taking Prozac. After some adjustments were made in the dosage, we noticed his anxiety had begun to diminish. As it lessened, we began to expose him to small situations that had always been troublesome for him and which he had meticulously avoided his whole life. We gave him new skills to use in these situations.

He began to order his own food at Burger King. He ordered pizza over the telephone, then went into the pizzeria with his mother, and eventually alone, to pick it up. He rode on escalators, went through revolving doors, talked to a teacher when he had a school problem, and bought school lunches and ate them. He returned an item to customer service at Target, and he joined the chess club at school. He couldn't do any of these things initially, but slowly learned how to do these tasks and many others. He even attended a one-week computer camp one summer, although he wouldn't sleep over. The next year he did stay at the camp overnight for a week. The following year, he stayed for two weeks and then finally five weeks, his last summer before high school graduation. He went to college away from home, shared a room with another student, and interacted with other students during some of his free time. He couldn't do everything equally well, nor did he become a "party animal." Rather, he became a more rounded young man who did not always allow anxiety to determine what he did. He could do new and different things when he planned them in advance. He stayed at college, achieved good grades, had a small social life, continued to have reduced anxiety, showed some flexibility, and even seemed to enjoy many of his new experiences. His parents didn't stop worrying about him. That never happens. They would always worry, but they also had hope that the skills they had given him would help him not just survive, but thrive. And, after all, isn't that what we always wanted?

Success for you and your child won't look the same as it does for someone else. You must never give up or become discouraged, even though you will be tempted. Your patience will be tried, your nerves will be frayed, and you'll be at your wit's end—but if you follow the ideas in our book, find a professional or two to help you, and don't become overwhelmed, you too will have success to write about.

10

Teaching the Asperger Student

HOW TO CREATE AN EFFECTIVE SCHOOL PROGRAM

Will entered my kindergarten class after a very unsuccessful preschool experience. He was described by his teachers as "out of control" on a daily basis and it was made clear he was not welcome to return the next year. There had been no successful interventions to modify or control his behavior. When all efforts, including individual supervision, had failed to help him get his behavior under control, his parents were called to pick him up. As the year progressed, he was spending less and less time in school. After reading Will's file and talking with his parents, I knew he would profit from the structure and consistency of my classroom. From his first day in my class, he did not display many of the problematic behaviors that had been reported, due to the high level of structure he was now receiving. However, Will continued to be very rigid and controlling, and these issues were addressed over the next two years.

The consistency of the classroom environment reduced his anxiety, which allowed me to introduce him to alternative and less rigid behaviors. The concepts of flexibility, problems and solutions, being okay, and good choice/bad choice were all introduced. As Will was able to successfully use these strategies, I began to sabotage his environment so that he could practice using them in situations that were more "real world." Remember, creating a specialized environment for the Asperger student is only the first step. This step decreases the student's anxiety and provides you with the opportunity to begin to teach alternative and more appropriate behaviors. The next, and most important, step is introducing change and challenges into his environment (planned sabotage) so that the student can generalize these skills and begin to function successfully in the larger world.

These steps were carefully followed with Will, and he was gradually mainstreamed without support into a typical first-grade classroom from my self-contained Asperger classroom. When he was ready to enter second grade, he did so without any specialized support. Will's experience provides an example of the type of progress that can be made when an Asperger child is placed in the appropriate setting. Because Will's intellectual and verbal skills were intact (academic skills were never a difficulty for him), he was able to learn alternative coping strategies that would allow him to be successful in school. The best summary of this experience comes from Will's own words. On the last day of school I ask each student if they would like to talk about their school year and what they have learned. Will had just completed first grade and knew he would not be returning to our program or school. This is what he said to the class: "When I came to this class two years ago I had a lot of questions. Who? What? Why? How? I didn't know how to answer these questions. I wanted to answer these questions. Now I know the answers. I know who, what, why, and how. That makes me feel good. I know the answers."

We had given Will alternative behaviors to handle frustrations and new strategies to use when feeling anxious or confused. In other words, Will had a plan, the road map. He now not only knew what to do, but how to do it. This is what he and all individuals with Asperger's syndrome need and want. How is this achieved in the school environment? What does an exemplary school program for the Asperger student look like? What are the core components of such a program? Let's explore the answers to these questions.

Essentials for a School Program

Any classroom environment should be designed to meet the needs of the learners in that classroom. This becomes crucial when the learner also has Asperger's syndrome. When working with the Asperger student you must be a choreographer, orchestrating many variables simultaneously. Successful interventions are built on a detailed understanding of each student and a clear analysis of what is needed. Broad, general cookie-cutter approaches will not be successful. CSIT emphasizes prevention, rather than consequences, to foster appropriate responses. You must create a classroom environment that is structured and firm, but flexible. It has to be predictable, while introducing change at the same time. This is accomplished by using step-by-step direct teaching with visuals to enhance learning as well as the teaching of coping strategies to reduce anxiety.

The consistent message you should be sending to the student is: "Change and challenges will happen: there are ways to deal with them, and I will teach you how to do that." A good program choreographs three levels of intervention: basic—developing and modifying strategies in order to obtain stability and prevent difficulties; advanced—developing generalization strategies while expanding the student's own repertoires; and crisis intervention—using challenges to teach more appropriate responding in the future. This will be achieved by focusing on the following techniques:

- The direct teaching of social thinking and social skills
- The direct teaching of flexibility and coping strategies for anxiety, which are the prevention strategies that will enable the student to cope with change
- The direct teaching of language and conversational skills
- The modification of special interests, rigidity, and routines
- Academic instruction based on the special needs of the Asperger student

Obviously, these techniques will be implemented in a different manner in a typical classroom, as opposed to a self-contained classroom. In addition, not all Asperger children have the same needs, nor do those needs remain consistent over time. You need to determine the correct strategy for a particular student at a particular time; this is important for success. Let's examine the components of an ideal core program, beginning with the attitude and personality you need to adopt when interacting with an Asperger child.

The Teacher's Personality

Your personality and how you use it to interact with the Asperger student is critical. The initial "face" you present to the student is the same as the one you will want in all of your permanent interactions with the student. Being "easy" or giving the student a "break" will undermine your ability to be a sphere of influence and thus will hinder his progress. Your behavior and style should follow the "Eight Guidelines for the Teacher" in the list below.

EIGHT GUIDELINES FOR THE TEACHER

1. Never miss an opportunity to be reinforcing or give praise, but do not give false praise.

2. Always, always, always be consistent in word and action. You will need to make rules and stick to them. When you make a request, you must always follow through. You do not make second requests and you do not plead. Choose your battles carefully because you cannot back down once you have made a request.

3. Always remember that the Asperger student is anxious and he should be able to look to you for security. Therefore, you must be in control at all times. The student needs to know that you are available to help him. You must convey to the student approaching a challenge that you will not allow him to escape the challenge, but he can depend upon you to help him complete the challenge.

4. Keep your language simple and consistent. In doing so, you will be able to provide the student with a "road map" to guide him

through interactions that he has trouble comprehending. Almost all new situations will need to be explained and modeled for the student. He will need to be told exactly what he can and cannot do.

5. Always remain on topic when involved in an interaction with the student. This is especially important during a crisis. At these times, the student will work hard to bring up extraneous or unrelated issues to try to justify his behavior or as an alternative to solving his problem. All such conversation must be ignored. You can state, "That's off topic; I can't talk about that," or "That does not make sense; I can't talk about that," or "That is not what we are talking about."

6. Always remain calm. If you do raise your voice, it is because you have planned to do so to make a particular point. This would most likely be during a modeling or role-playing activity and certainly not during a crisis.

7. You must be able to determine when the student begins to get anxious so that you can intervene early, before it escalates.

8. Create a structured environment and follow a set routine. You must be very organized, but at the same time very flexible.

A Proper Assessment

All of the individuals responsible for the student's program must be knowledgeable about Asperger's syndrome, otherwise they won't understand the subtleties that motivate the child's behavior. A proper assessment needs to look beyond the usual areas (academic levels, task completion, direction following) if it is to fulfill its crucial role of determining which strategies to select. Our assessments focus on understanding behavior. The questions in the sidebar provide a guide of what you need to be looking for as you observe the student. The data from the observations will enable you to decide what behaviors need to be changed or eliminated.

QUESTIONS FOR BEHAVIORAL OBSERVATION

1. How does the student use unstructured time?

2. How does the student interact with peers? with adults?

3. How does the student use language to communicate?

4. How does the student exert control over his environment?

5. Does the student use reciprocal language in social interactions?

6. Does the student attempt to control language exchanges? If so, how is this done?

7. Does the student use language scripts?

8. Does the student have special fears, obsessions, or fixations?

9. Does the student have control issues?

10. Do patterns, routines, rituals, or rigidity interfere with the student's functioning? If so, how does the student react when these are disrupted?

11. How does the student respond to frustration?

12. How does the student respond to change?

13. What is the student's degree of noncompliance? How is it manifested?

14. What type of sensory issues does the student display? How are they manifested?

In making these observations, you need to look beneath the surface behavior. Once you have selected behaviors to change or eliminate, you must determine what motivates the behavior. Only then can you begin to design effective intervention strategies that will focus upon teaching new skills. Success will depend upon you or the team you are working with having the ability and resources to modify the environment based on the results. It is imperative that your strategies be based on the student's needs and not on a fixed method. It is also crucial to match strategies to the Asperger subtype of the child or teen as discussed in chapter 3.

A Consistent and Predictable Environment

The initial goal is to create an environment where the student feels comfortable. The environment is a combination of the classroom's physical space and the rules you institute. Both will be characterized by consistency, so that how you structure the room's space and present your rules will support the teaching environment. A structured and consistent environment will relieve the student's anxiety and allow him to be more open to change and/or challenges. As he begins to understand the interactions around him, he will begin to feel competent. The sidebars below and on pages 212–213 contain guidelines for both parts of the environment.

Skill-Centered Interventions and Teaching

Skill-centered intervention techniques focus on giving the student skills he can use to succeed. These are very different from intervention models that depend upon redirection or prompting—their goal is simply establishing control and compliance. Skill-centered models, on the other hand, help to expand your child's repertoire by teaching new skills—skills that will help him to be independent. Among the many aspects to address in

GUIDELINES FOR THE CLASSROOM'S PHYSICAL SPACE

1. *Provide a classroom space that has physical consistency.* Changes shouldn't be made unless you have carefully planned for them.

2. *Identify consistent areas in the classroom for specific activities.* These should be associated with consistent behavioral expectations for those activities.

3. *Provide clearly labeled materials* and make clear which materials are accessible to the student and which are not.

4. *Initially assign seating,* but plan for random seating in the future.

5. *Provide visually clear boundaries* for different areas in the room.

GUIDELINES FOR REDUCING STUDENT ANXIETY

1. *Provide routine, structure, consistency, and predictability,* but remember structure does not mean a rigid environment.

2. *Minimize transitions* initially and always plan for them.

3. *When using a reward/consequence system, make sure it is clearly explained and understood* by the student. Know what the student views as a reward or consequence. These are often unusual for the Asperger student, so your system will need to be individualized. Using natural consequences and having preferred activities follow nonpreferred activities are most beneficial.

4. *Provide "structured teaching"*—structure the activity, the interaction, and the environment. All teaching is provided in a definite pattern of organization to establish clear patterns, so that the student can anticipate what will be next. You will teach activities not typically taught to students whose cognitive functioning is average or above (how to walk in the hallway; use the school bathroom; take back a lunch tray; and unpack and pack a school bag). Teaching must be step by step and should use visuals.

5. *Teach that rules can have "shades of gray" very early.* Practice this.

6. *Use role-playing of both appropriate and inappropriate behaviors.* Be sure to practice these skills with problems occurring (someone is standing in front of your cubby or locker; you forgot the combination of your locker; the bathroom is crowded; a person bumps into you in the cafeteria).

7. *Always interrupt inappropriate language* (repeating jokes too often, exaggerated or nonsense stories, stories that go on too long, speaking like an animal or imaginary character) and model examples of appropriate language.

8. *Use written scripts* to assist the student and circumvent his difficulty with language.

9. *When teaching replacement behaviors* use visual and verbal prompts, modeling, role-playing, guided practice, rehearsal, social stories, natural consequences, problems and solutions, and good choice/bad choice.

10. *Set a daily routine.* The opening activity should present the day's schedule. Use this to discuss and plan for even the most minor changes (especially in the beginning—remember, this is a prevention model).

continued

GUIDELINES FOR REDUCING STUDENT ANXIETY
cont'd

11. *Remember, once a routine or rule is established, it will be difficult to change.* Use sabotage and teach flexibility.

12. *Develop key words and phrases* that can act as cues (verbal prompts are a step along the way to self-prompting and independence).

13. *All new learning should be presented using a visual hierarchy of prompts:* picture instruction; hand cues; cue cards; posting schedules, rules, and key phrases; marking physical boundaries with masking tape.

14. *Posted rules should be clear and brief.* Involve the student in rule formation—the feeling of having some control helps reduce the anxiety.

15. *Be aware of sensory issues.* If any sensitivity-based behaviors no longer apply—they've become mere habit—treat them as you would any other inappropriate behavior.

16. *Teach the student to observe peers very early and use them as social cues.*

support of these core skills are a child's language and academic needs, as well as issues surrounding perfectionism, blending in with peers, and staying focused.

ADDRESSING SPECIALIZED LANGUAGE NEEDS

A part of your child's independence will depend on her ability to communicate with others through language. Unfortunately, appropriate use of language is very difficult for the Asperger child. She may have one-sided conversations with others about her interests—with seemingly no awareness that her listeners aren't interested. Or she may follow repetitive scripts that don't support the normal back-and-forth flow of conversations. Whatever the case, teaching language skills that allow the Asperger student to communicate with the world around her has to be a part of any core curriculum. Improving language processing, comprehension, and expression will improve behaviors in the same way a more structured environment will improve behavior. Below are the guidelines and skills that need to be a part of the child's language program.

1. Language learning should occur all day (and every day) in context, as it happens. Use naturally occurring language "events," such as the child's difficulty coping with a change in the schedule, to teach appropriate language.

2. Use consistent language and gestures and initially pair them with visuals. The development of key words and phrases will be crucial (key words and phrases will only be effective if you have demonstrated exactly what they mean and then use them consistently).

3. Post or write on cue cards key words, phrases, or gestures.

4. In general, keep your voice calm and even, though at times you will have to be overly dramatic to improve the student's ability to "read" emotional expression.

5. Avoid too much praise, so that perfectionism is not inadvertently reinforced.

6. Teach language scripts, but remember these are only guides to help the student start. Interrupt predetermined language scripts that the student may use.

7. Reflect back when a student misinterprets a situation and label it correctly for him.

8. Label and limit obsessive or off-topic talking.

9. Directly teach correct tone and volume. Give the reason for why these skills are needed; do not simply teach the skill.

10. Directly teach nonverbal communication skills (eye gaze, body posture, use of gestures, facial expression, personal space). Do not simply teach the skill; explain why these skills are necessary.

11. Teach all aspects of conversational language (e.g., initiation, maintenance, and conclusion of conversations; taking turns in conversations; the use of questions and comments; topic maintenance).

12. Directly teach the appropriate use of "I don't know" and "I need help." The Asperger student has great difficulty with these responses.

13. Always avoid vague directions and nonspecific language; for example, do not say "Raise your hand," but instead, "Before you speak, raise your hand and wait for the teacher to say your name."

14. Use consistent phrases when giving directions; for example, "Tell me what you need to do," "Show me that you can _____," "Show me what [a certain activity] looks like." "I see that you are _____."

15. Use examples, not explanations—say, "This is how school sitting looks," or "This is how we walk in the hall," then demonstrate.

16. Label new tasks or activities as difficult, to reduce student anxiety: "This is hard; no one gets this right the first time."

ADDRESSING ACADEMIC NEEDS

Learning academic material requires expertise in a number of secondary skill areas, from organization to coping with frustrating assignments. The list below outlines these skills and guidelines for the teacher to follow:

1. Use direct teaching of organizational skills that are necessary to learning.

2. Provide for generalization of all new skills learned. It is helpful to use a thematic approach, integrated into the curriculum, to foster generalization and organization. Try to keep teaching strategies similar across situations, so that when presenting new material you are able to point out the similarities or connections to past material.

3. Focus on the teaching of abstract skills in all academic areas. When teaching abstract skills use a hands-on approach whenever

possible. For instance, when studying volcanoes, actually build and erupt a model.

4. Teach reading as visually as possible. Use Venn diagrams, word webs, attribute webs, mind maps, and cartoons. Remember, word recognition and oral reading will often be strong, whereas comprehension will be lagging or nonexistent. Reading should be taught at the student's comprehension level.

5. Teach math as visually as possible by using manipulatives. Teach the math vocabulary needed for a specific math skill prior to introducing the skill.

6. Teach handwriting in a very structured step-by-step approach. Use writing in blocks and colored lines, describe the formation of each individual letter or number, and use key words and phrases to describe the process of letter and number writing ("*L* is a tall letter, so it needs to bump the top and bottom line" or "Small letter *a* is a circle with a line"). Be aware that some handwriting difficulties may be due to the Asperger student's own high standards and perfectionism issues.

7. Instructions should be simple and clear. Allow the student to repeat to you what they have to do. Use visuals.

DEALING WITH PERFECTIONISM

Many behaviors displayed by Asperger children are often misinterpreted, a common one being their sense of perfectionism. Some teachers may see the child's perfectionism as the child simply working hard to do his best. However, perfectionism is just one of many ways the Asperger student tries to control his world and anxiety. He sees the world in black-and-white terms. Either he is perfect or what he does is horrible; there is no in between. In the long run, the rigidity and inflexibility of perfectionism will lead to greater anxiety and more problems. It is important for you to combat this. You need to downplay perfect papers; children need to see their mistakes as part of the normal learning process. The Asperger student needs to learn that there are "shades of gray" with regard to task quality. Some ways you can do this are to act as a model by making mistakes yourself and pointing them out, to encourage the use of invented spelling (this is very difficult for the Asperger student, but it will increase his flexibility), to label a task as being hard (as opposed to labeling the student's attempt as a failure), to limit erasing, and finally to reward *the effort* rather than perfection.

HELPING THE STUDENT TO BLEND IN

At the other end of the spectrum, there are those behaviors and interests that mark the Asperger student as different. Many of these are not academic, but it is important to help the Asperger student to reduce or eliminate these behaviors so that he can blend in successfully with peers. It is important to note that these special interests or eccentricities are not expressions of independence and individuality. Rather, they reflect the ways the child copes with his anxiety and his difficulty understanding social cues. They are not choices. It is your job as the teacher to improve the student's blending in by helping him to independently perform self-help skills typical of same-age peers (dressing, grooming, eating, going to the bathroom); engage in school skills typical of same-age peers (using a book bag, buying lunch, riding the bus); and make age-appropriate selections in terms of clothes, accessories, play and leisure choices, and music/TV/book/movie/game choices. Doing this will decrease anxiety and increase independent functioning.

KEEPING THE STUDENT FOCUSED

Finally, be aware of distractibility issues. The Asperger student is a master of tuning out the external environment to be in his own world. To help maintain the student's attention, you should:

1. Present materials visually.

2. Use a thematic or hands-on teaching style to increase student engagement.

3. Clarify what constitutes the start and finish of a task.

4. Control and use the student's special interests to gain attention in an activity.

5. Use visual organizers (schedules, assignment sheets, planning charts, checklists, color-coded file folders, etc.).

USING A REWARD SYSTEM

In working on all the issues discussed here and elsewhere in the book, remember to incorporate a reward system. The Asperger student will display a restricted range of interests that serves a variety of purposes for him (facilitating conversation, providing a feeling of competence, relieving anxiety, providing order and consistency, providing relaxation and enjoyment). You can use these interests as rewards. To do this, you must limit and control access to the interest (designate the amount of time that can be spent on the interest and where it can be done, such as limiting Internet time or the amount of time spent discussing an interest). The interest can then be used as a reward for completing a less desirable task. When possible, incorporate the interests into teaching strategies, which then provide the student with appropriate ways to engage in the activity. Used in this way, the interest becomes a "draw" to learn a less interesting skill. You will be using a narrow interest as a way to expand the student's repertoire and activities.

Prevention and Sabotage

You should use prevention strategies as much as possible. When using prevention strategies, the techniques and language used must be practiced over and over. The strategies build upon one another and using them together will create understanding and encourage generalization. This will mean anticipating problems and practicing with the student before the event or crisis occurs. Your goal is to teach—in a step-by-step manner—coping skills and alternate behaviors as alternatives to the inappropriate behaviors the student has been using.

An important part of this process will be the gradual and systematic sabotaging of the environment to expose the student to change and to the realities of the world at large. This will further increase the student's feelings of competence and his ability to act independently in an unpredictable environment. As the environment is sabotaged the student will need fewer and fewer modifications to interact. He will be able to handle more and more typical situations without prompts.

Once the student's initial comfort level has been established, you can begin to introduce the planned changes of your sabotage effort on a daily basis. It is important to introduce and reward change on a regular basis. The daily goal is to systematically decrease rigidity and increase flexibility. This is the only way to guarantee generalization and permanent change. For some students, this can begin as a very small change (trying a different brand of juice), and for others, a larger change (playing ball with a new student on the playground). How quickly you move and the amount of change you attempt needs to be individualized for each student. Making some regular change, however small, should occur for all students.

The end result of prevention and sabotage will be increased flexibility in your student. With this skill under his belt, he is ready to face yet another challenge: mainstreaming.

Mainstreaming Techniques

When you are ready to begin mainstreaming a student with Asperger's syndrome, it will need to be accomplished slowly and systematically in order for it to be successful. We see this as a two-step process, beginning with supervised mainstreaming and ending with unsupervised mainstreaming. Depending on the needs of the particular student and the skill of the school staff, this phase could last anywhere from two months to two years. Let's look at what is involved in each step of this process.

Step 1: Supervised Mainstreaming

Your first task is to observe the mainstream setting to determine the social, behavioral, language, and academic skills the student will need when he leaves his specialized class.

Next, the receiving teacher should be provided with some general knowledge of Asperger's syndrome and then specific details concerning the student to be mainstreamed. This would include: learning issues, social difficulties, any obsessive-compulsive/rigidity/control issues, and how to recognize anxiety. My self-contained class is mainstreamed as a whole each day into a regular class, accompanied by both the teacher and the assistant. This allows the regular teacher to observe and become familiar with my students—long before any unsupervised mainstreaming would occur. She is able to witness firsthand the strategies and techniques that are successful, rather than just hear or read about them. In addition, it allows the Asperger student to become familiar with the teacher, her teaching techniques, her teaching style, her students, and the general flow of that classroom. He has the "road map," or "game plan," and knows what will be expected. This will immediately lower his anxiety about attending the class without support. Providing the Asperger student with this type of mainstream experience is ideal.

Even with supervised mainstreaming, it will be important to initially pick those activities where the Asperger student can be the most successful. Nonacademic subjects (library, music, art—but not gym) tend to be the least stressful. In elementary school, science and/or social studies, because they are often presented in a hands-on, visual style, would be appropriate. Avoid activities that involve a lot of cooperative learning, abstract skills, and writing. Instead, try to pick academic areas that are strengths for the Asperger student.

Step 2: Unsupervised Mainstreaming

Ideally, the move to unsupervised mainstreaming starts in a classroom where supervised mainstreaming has already occurred. Initially, mainstreaming should be brief (a half hour in elementary school, up to one hour in high school), and in a strength area for that particular student. When the student demonstrates success with this first activity, gradually add other activities. Avoid adding more than one new activity at a time. Initially, each new class added should be for a brief period.

If seats are assigned be very careful regarding the particular students the Asperger student sits near. They should be successful students, without behavior issues, who are able to act as models or give guidance. Often, the Asperger student will look to others when he is unsure of what to do; however, rather than ask for help, he may copy what another is doing. This is a good strategy. I regularly tell my students, "If you do not know what to do, look at the students around you and do what they are doing."

When they are unable to model independently, they may take verbal advice offered by another student, "Don't forget to put your name on your paper" or "We have to use a red crayon." Clustering student desks in groups of four makes a large classroom more organized and provides the Asperger student with a consistent and small group of students for him to interact with. Again, in this way the Asperger student will have a group of students to use as cues to determine if he is working on the correct task, using the correct materials, working at the correct speed, and behaving as the other students are. The students should be able to offer help, but not too much. They should be talkative (to encourage back-and-forth conversation), but not too talkative.

The regular teacher will need to make modifications. These might include:

- Using cue cards

- Providing more classroom visuals

- Making use of previously taught key words and phrases

- Using consistent and clear language

- Providing advance warning of transitions

• Checking with the Asperger student to make sure directions have been understood, as they may not ask for help ("Tell me what you have to do.")

• Providing special seating for the Asperger student

• Providing an individual schedule for the Asperger student

• Periodically meeting with the Asperger student to clearly explain the classroom rules/routine/expectations, as these can change over time. Developing a special cue between the Asperger student and teacher to signal inappropriate behaviors will be important. The more structured and consistent the classroom can be, the less anxious the Asperger student will be. This will decrease inappropriate behaviors, increase focusing, and allow the student to practice new skills.

As mainstreaming increases to include less structured activities (such as lunch or recess), someone will need to monitor these activities to make sure the Asperger student is able to appropriately engage with others. A good idea is to provide the Asperger student with a "buddy" during these periods. This buddy could help to provide awareness of the social cues that the Asperger student often misses.

Most likely, some additional skills training will need to be provided by the special education teacher. The special education teacher will need to be available to the regular teacher on a daily basis to provide support for problems that may arise. In addition, the special education teacher will continue to provide support to the Asperger student. This might include:

• Developing social stories, cue cards, new key words or phrases, and organizational strategies

• Providing additional skills development in the areas of flexibility and planned sabotage

• Teaching anxiety-reducing techniques and coping strategies

● Providing additional development in the areas of social thinking and social skills

● Providing crisis intervention

● Preparing and practicing with the Asperger student for upcoming novel activities and skills that will be presented in the regular classroom

● Providing the Asperger student with additional support in academic areas. Giving the Asperger student "sneak previews" prior to the introduction of new materials or activities is crucial. Remember, someone will still need to be teaching new skills and monitoring old ones. In other words, support is needed.

If the unsupervised mainstreaming will not be occurring in the same building as the supervised mainstreaming or if the student is ready to move to another school building (such as one closer to his home), it will be important that at least one member of the new educational staff is knowledgeable concerning Asperger's syndrome. This staff member will need to develop a relationship with the student immediately, so they can act as a resource when difficulties arise. Ideally, all teachers working with the student with Asperger's syndrome should be provided with training.

Inclusion Techniques

Some Asperger children or teens will receive all of their special education services in the regular classroom rather than a self-contained or resource room. This is called *inclusion*. Helping children and teens in inclusion is difficult because there may not be anyone overseeing their program. Ideally, all individuals working with the student should be trained in the nature of Asperger's syndrome: key concepts, intervention strategies, skill development, and crisis prevention. We have found that three full days are required to adequately train staff. Even with this, there needs to be periodic follow-ups to review progress.

To ensure that problems don't get out of hand, team meetings with all concerned parties should occur on a regular basis to evaluate progress and redefine goals as necessary. To stay on top of problems and to be responsible for calling such meetings, someone on staff should be appointed as the "case manager."

Prior to the beginning of the day, the student should report to the person designated to act as the case manager. The case manager's role is to ensure that all Individualized Education Program (IEP) goals are being delivered and to monitor the student's progress. The case manager will check on the materials and work assignments needed for the day, as well as discuss any issues from the previous day, develop strategies, and review any other pertinent matters.

At the secondary grade level, the student needs to have a home room, and will go to it at the designated time. A schedule of classes will be developed that reflects the student's ability in each subject. At some time during the day there will be a resource room class where any academic, social, or behavioral needs will be taught or reinforced. This should be scheduled at least once a day for a specific time. At the end of the day, the student once again meets with the case manager to repeat what occurred in the morning. All teachers during the day will issue reports on the student for the case manager to review. If any problems are revealed, further follow-up may be necessary, which may involve, for example, the case manager sitting in on selected classes.

At least once per week, there should be a social skills lesson, or counseling session, to discuss at greater length any issues that are recurring and/or to work on social or behavioral skills development.

Contingency Accommodations

IEP goals should be created that have *contingency accommodations*, because it is not always clear when specially designed instruction will be necessary. In keeping with this, you should create a list of accommodations and modifications that might be necessary if concerns arise. Some of these accommodations would be:

- Extra time to complete assignments

- Alternate, more concrete assignments instead of those that are abstract

- Shorter assignments—fewer problems to do, fewer spelling words, fewer sentences, etc.

- Copies of notes from the teacher or another student

- Short-answer test questions instead of essay questions

- Additional explanations of assignments to check on comprehension

- Opportunities to correct or redo assignments with parental support

- Verbal completion of tests or assignments if written responses are a problem

As the child moves through school, there will be many issues that will need to be addressed. These issues increase as the middle school and high school years approach. Foremost among these issues are organization skills. Keeping track of homework, projects, and long-term assignments is very difficult for Asperger students. In middle school and high school, there are concerns involving lockers, the use of a six-day schedule or "A" and "B" days, and managing papers and materials from each class.

There are also difficulties that arise from specific types of assignments, specifically those involving abstract concepts such as opinions, feelings, and comparisons, and any other assignments that involve higher order thinking. You will have to teach the student how to make a choice when one has no opinion—for example, by flipping a coin. The student may need help in answering questions such as, "Tell us why you liked one of the two stories we read." For this, we have to create an algorithm providing the student with a structure to arrive at an answer. For example, you could create a checklist like the one in the sidebar on page 226.

Though the guidelines mentioned above are crucial for successfully

SAMPLE STRUCTURE TO HELP A STUDENT DECIDE WHICH STORY HE OR SHE PREFERS AND WHY

To the student say, "Make a list indicating whether you liked or disliked each of the following points for each story read":

	Story 1	Story 2
1. Characters in the story	Liked	Disliked
2. Length of the story	Liked	Liked
3. Vocabulary in the story	Disliked	Disliked
4. How interesting was the story	Liked	Liked
5. Would you read it again?	Yes	No

"As a result, it looks like you liked Story 1 more and the reasons are indicated above." This would then be written up in narrative format to answer the question of which story the student liked better.

mainstreaming an Asperger student, one element remains the most critical for success: the receptiveness of the staff receiving the student. Their ability to understand him and make the appropriate modifications makes all the difference.

Parental Involvement

A program's success will be limited if the teacher can't build a trusting and strong connection with the parents. Prior to her initial involvement with the student, the teacher will need to meet with his family so that she can get a clearer picture of the student's needs and begin to formulate a plan for how to assist the family in generalizing new skills outside of the classroom. This is also a time to begin to discuss with the student's family the types of strategies the teacher will be using and how the parents can learn to use these strategies at home. (Use the "Parent Questionnaire" in appendix E.)

Parents and teachers need to be aware of and be able to consistently use the coping strategies, key words and phrases, and prevention strategies that are used in the classroom. Without this, generalization will be limited. In elementary school, communication should be on a daily basis and can be provided through a copybook that can travel back and forth between home and school. As the student enters middle school, a weekly phone call would probably suffice.

If the teacher is knowledgeable about working with Asperger children, planned changes and sabotage should be completed within the school setting before the home. Because the Asperger student has no prior history with the teacher, the process should be smoother. Once this is achieved at school, you can begin to plan for generalization at home. Parents may need significant demonstration of strategies and support from the teacher at these times. If the parents are more knowledgeable than the teacher, she might need their help on how to makes changes using sabotage.

Besides IEP reviews and progress reports, there should be a way to determine if the student's needs, both at home and school, have been met. An "End-of-Year Evaluation" form is included in appendix F as one way in which to achieve this goal.

We have worked with parents for more than twenty-five years and believe that the ability of professionals and parents to work together effectively is a significant determinant of student success. The teaching of an Asperger student cannot remain isolated within the classroom. To achieve successful generalization, school will have to venture into the student's home (figuratively). It will be impossible to do this without fostering a school/home bond. Professionals must ensure that each student meets realistic goals in both current and future development. We take wisdom from the Duchess in *Alice in Wonderland,* who says to Alice, "Be who you are, or if you would like it put more simply, never try to be what you might have been or could have been, other than what you should have been." We will not be able to do this if parents and professionals are not on the same team.

APPENDIX A

Characteristics Checklist for Asperger's Syndrome

This appendix contains a description of the characteristics displayed by children and teens with Asperger's syndrome. Once again, because our approach is practical, we provide descriptions of the characteristics, rather than merely listing them. By describing what a particular characteristic will look like when displayed, you will have a clearer picture of which characteristics are most problematic for your child. Before you begin to work on problems, you must know what those problems are and how they are manifested.

The characteristic list is presented in a checklist format. We encourage you to copy this checklist and share it with all those involved with your child. It will be useful in determining initial diagnosis. Later, it will help those working with your child to better understand how particular attributes are translated into behaviors. The result will be a clearer understanding of the reasons behind the behaviors displayed by your child. It is important to remember that the more you understand about Asperger behaviors and the reasons behind them, the more effective you will be when you begin to intervene and change behaviors.

When completing this checklist, check off all characteristics that apply to your child. Use the examples given as illustrations. Some characteristics overlap with others, so don't worry. Moreover, a characteristic should still be checked, even if it doesn't occur all of the time. Your child may display the same behavior, or he may exhibit his own particular variation. He may be an individual with Asperger's syndrome, but he remains an individual.

I. DIFFICULTY WITH RECIPROCAL SOCIAL INTERACTIONS

A. Inability and/or a lack of desire to interact with peers. You are concerned with the child's reciprocal interactions with others and the quality of those interactions. It is very important to observe how the child interacts with same-age peers. This category comprises two separate issues: the ability and the desire to interact.

☐ **1.** Displays an *inability* to interact because she does not know how to interact. She wants to interact with others but does not know what to do.

☐   **a.** Observes or stays on the periphery of a group rather than joining in

☐   **b.** Initiates play interaction by taking a toy or starting to engage in an ongoing activity without gaining verbal agreement from the other players, will ignore a negative response from others when asking to join in, will abruptly leave a play interaction

☐   **c.** Lacks conversational language for a social purpose, does not know what to say—this could be no conversation, monopolizing the conversation, lack of ability to initiate conversation, obsessive conversation in one area, conversation not on topic or conversation that is not of interest to others

☐   **d.** Lacks the ability to understand, attend to, maintain, or repair a conversational flow or exchange—this causes miscommunication and inappropriate responses (unable to use the back-and-forth aspect of communication)

☐   **e.** Lacks an understanding of game playing—unable to share, unable to follow the rules of turn taking, unable to follow game-playing rules (even those that may appear quite obvious), is rigid in game playing (may want to control the game or those playing and/or create her own set of rules), always needs to be first, unable to make appropriate comments while playing, and has difficulty with winning/losing

☐   **f.** Is unable to select activities that are of interest to others (unaware or unconcerned that others do not share the same interest or level of interest, unable to compromise)

☐   **g.** Compromises interactions by rigidity, inability to shift attention or "go with the flow," being rule bound, needs to control the play/activity (play may "look" imaginative but is most likely repetitive—e.g., action figures are always used in the same way, songs are played in the same order, Lego pieces are always put together in the same way)

☐   **h.** Displays narrow play and activity choices (best observed during unstructured play/leisure activities: look for rigidity/patterns/repetitive choices, inability to accept novelty)

☐   **i.** Engages in unusual behaviors or activities (selects play or activity choices of a younger child, seems unaware of the unwritten social rules among peers, acts like an imaginary character, uses an unusual voice—any behaviors that call attention to the individual or are viewed as unusual by peers)

☐   **j.** Displays a limited awareness of current fashion, slang, topics, activities, and accessories (does not seem interested in what peers view as popular or the most current craze, unless it happens to match a special interest)

☐   **k.** Displays a limited awareness of the emotions of others and/or how to respond to them (does not ask for help from others, does not know how to respond when help is given, does not know how to respond to compliments, does not realize the importance of apologizing, does not realize something she says or does can hurt the feelings of another, does not differentiate internal thoughts from external thoughts, does not respond to the emotions another is displaying—misses cues)

☐   **l.** Prefers structured over nonstructured activities

☐ **2.** Displays a *lack of desire* to interact.

☐   **a.** Does not care about her inability to interact with others because she has no interest in doing so. She prefers solitary activities and does not have the need to interact with others, or she is socially indifferent and can take it or leave it with regard to interacting with others.

☐   **b.** Sits apart from others, avoids situations where involvement with others is expected (playgrounds, birthday parties, being outside in general), and selects activities that are best completed alone (e.g., computer games, Game Boy, books, viewing TV/videos, collecting, keeping lists).

☐   **c.** Is rule bound/rigid and spends all free time completely consumed by areas of special interest. Her activities are so rule bound, it would be almost impossible for a peer to join in correctly. When asked about preferred friends, the individual is unable to name any or names those who are really not friends (family members, teachers).

B. Lack of appreciation of social cues. The individual, unable to identify or interpret the "messages" others give in conversations or interactions, demonstrates social thinking deficits.

❑ **1.** Lacks awareness if someone appears bored, upset, angry, scared, and so forth. Therefore, she does not comment in a socially appropriate manner or respond by modifying the interaction.

❑ **2.** Lacks awareness of the facial expressions and body language of others, so these conversational cues are missed. He is also unable to use gestures or facial expressions to convey meaning when conversing. You will see fleeting, averted, or a lack of eye contact. He will fail to gain another's attention before conversing with them. He may stand too far away from or too close to the person he is conversing with. His body posture may appear unusual.

❑ **3.** When questioned regarding what could be learned from another's facial expression, says, "Nothing." Faces do not provide him with information. Unable to read these "messages," he is unable to respond to them.

❑ **4.** Has difficulty with feelings of empathy for others. Interactions with others remain on one level, with one message.
❑　　**a.** Ignores an individual's appearance of sadness, anger, boredom, etc.
❑　　**b.** Fails to assist someone with an obvious need for help (not holding a door for someone carrying many items or assisting someone who falls or drops their belongings)
❑　　**c.** Talks on and on about a special interest while unaware that the other person is no longer paying attention, talks to someone who is obviously engaged in another activity, talks to someone who isn't even there

C. Socially and emotionally inappropriate behaviors. This is a direct result of not understanding the rules of social interactions. If you don't understand what someone is saying or doing, you will be unable to give the appropriate response.

❑ 1. Laughs at something that is sad, asks questions that are too personal

❑ 2. Makes rude comments (tells someone they are fat, bald, old, have yellow teeth)

❑ 3. Engages in self-stimulatory or odd behaviors (rocking, tics, finger posturing, eye blinking, noises—humming/clicking/talking to self)

❑ 4. Is unaware of unspoken or "hidden" rules—may "tell" on peers, breaking the "code of silence" that exists. He will then be unaware why others are angry with him.

❑ 5. Responds with anger when he feels others are not following the rules, will discipline others or reprimand them for their actions (acts like the teacher or parent with peers)

❑ 6. Touches, hugs, or kisses others without realizing that it is inappropriate

D. Limited or abnormal use of nonverbal communication. The individual uses gestures, body language, or facial expressions infrequently or atypically when interacting with others.

❑ 1. Averts eye contact, or keeps it fleeting or limited

❑ 2. Stares intensely at people or objects

❑ 3. Does not observe personal space (is too close or too far)

❑ 4. Does not use gestures/body language when communicating

❑ **5.** Uses gestures/body language, but in an unusual manner

❑ **6.** Does not appear to comprehend the gestures/body language of others

❑ **7.** Uses facial expressions that do not match the emotion being expressed

❑ **8.** Lacks facial expressions when communicating

❑ **9.** Does not appear to comprehend the facial expressions of others

❑ **10.** Displays abnormal gestures/facial expressions/body posture when communicating. E.g.:
❑   **a.** Looks to the left or right of the person she is talking to
❑   **b.** Does not turn to face the person she is talking to
❑   **c.** Confronts another person without changing her face or voice
❑   **d.** Stands too close or too far away from another person
❑   **e.** Smiles when someone shares sad news
❑   **f.** Has tics or facial grimaces

II. IMPAIRMENTS IN LANGUAGE SKILLS

A. Impairment in the *pragmatic* use of language. This refers to the inability to use language in a social sense, as a way to interact/communicate with other people. It is important to observe the individual's use of language in various settings with various people (especially peers). Since the impairments are in pragmatic language usage, the individual will often score well on typical language tests. This does not mean his language is intact or that direct instruction, with opportunities for generalization, is not needed.

❑ **1.** Uses conversation to convey facts and information about special interests, rather than to convey thoughts, emotions, or feelings

❑ **2.** Uses language scripts or verbal rituals in conversation, often described as "nonsense talk" by others (scripts may be made up or taken from movies/books/TV). At times, the scripts are subtle and may be difficult to detect.

❑ **3.** Has difficulty initiating, maintaining, and ending conversations with others. E.g.:

❑   **a.** Focuses conversations on one narrow topic, with too many details given, or moves from one seemingly unrelated topic to the next

❑   **b.** Once a discussion begins it is as if there is no "stop" button; must complete a predetermined dialogue

❑   **c.** Knows how to make a greeting, but has no idea how to continue the conversation; the next comment may be one that is totally irrelevant

❑   **d.** Does not make conversations reciprocal (has great difficulty with the back-and-forth aspect), attempts to control the language exchange, may leave a conversation before it is concluded

❑   **e.** Does not inquire about others when conversing

❑ **4.** Is unsure how to ask for help/make requests/make comments.

❑   **a.** Fails to inquire regarding others

❑   **b.** Makes comments that may embarrass others

❑   **c.** Interrupts others

❑   **d.** Engages in obsessive questioning or talking in one area, lacks interest in the topics of others

❑   **e.** Has difficulty maintaining the conversation *topic*

B. Impairment in the *semantic* use of language. This refers to understanding the language being used.

❑ **1.** Displays difficulty understanding not only individual words, but conversations and materials that are read

❑ **2.** Displays difficulty with problem solving

❑ **3.** Displays difficulty analyzing/synthesizing information presented.

❑   **a.** Does not ask for the meaning of an unknown word

❑   **b.** Uses words in a peculiar manner

❑   **c.** Is unable to make or understand jokes/teasing

❑   **d.** Creates jokes that make no sense

❑   **e.** Interprets known words on a literal level (concrete thinking)

❑   **f.** Has a large vocabulary consisting mainly of nouns and verbs

❑   **g.** Creates own words, using them with great pleasure in social situations

❑   **h.** Has difficulty discriminating between fact and fantasy

C. **Impairment in *prosody*. This refers to the pitch, stress, and rhythm of an individual's voice.**

❑ **1.** Rarely varies the pitch, stress, rhythm, or melody of his speech. Does not realize this can convey meaning

❑ **2.** Has a voice pattern that is often described as robotic or as the "little professor"; in children, the rhythm of speech is more adultlike than childlike

❑ **3.** Displays difficulty with volume control (too loud or too soft)

❑ **4.** Uses the voice of a movie or cartoon character conversationally and is unaware that this is inappropriate

❑ **5.** Has difficulty understanding the meaning conveyed by others when they vary their pitch, rhythm, or tone

D. **Impairment in the *processing* of language. This refers to one's ability to comprehend what has been said. The Asperger individual has difficulty absorbing, analyzing, and then responding to the information.**

❑ **1.** When processing language (which requires multiple channels working together), has difficulty regulating just one channel, difficulty discriminating between relevant and irrelevant information

❑ **2.** Has difficulty shifting from one channel to another; processing is slow and easily interrupted by any environmental stimulation (seen as difficulty with topic maintenance). This will appear as distractibility or inattentiveness. (*Note:* When looking at focusing issues it is very difficult to determine the motivator. It could be attributed to one or a few of the following reasons: lack of interest, fantasy involvement, anxiety, or processing difficulty.)

❑ **3.** Displays a delay when answering questions

❑ **4.** Displays difficulty sustaining attention and is easily distracted (one might be discussing plants and the Asperger individual will ask a question about another country—something said may have triggered this connection or the individual may still be in an earlier conversation)

❑ **5.** Displays difficulty as language moves from a literal to a more abstract level (generalization difficulties found in the Asperger population are, in part, due to these processing difficulties)

III. NARROW RANGE OF INTERESTS AND INSISTENCE ON SET ROUTINES. THIS REFERS TO THE INDIVIDUAL'S RIGIDITY, OBSESSIONS, PERSEVERATIONS, AND NEED FOR STRUCTURE/ROUTINE/ORDER.

A. Rules are very important as the world is seen as black or white.

❑ **1.** Takes perfectionism to an extreme—one wrong answer is not tolerable and the individual must do things perfectly

❑ **2.** Has difficulty with any changes in the established routine

❑ **3.** Has a set routine for how activities are to be done

❑ **4.** Has rules for most activities, which must be followed (this can be extended to all involved)

B. The individual has few interests, but those present are unusual and treated as obsessions.

❑ **1.** Patterns, routines, and rituals are evident and interfere with daily functioning (this is driven by the individual's anxiety: the world is confusing for her, she is unsure what to do and how to do it—if she can impose structure she begins to have a feeling of control)

❑ **2.** Has developed narrow and specific interests; the interests tend to be atypical (this gives a feeling of competence and order). Involvement with the area of special interest becomes all-consuming.

❑ **3.** Displays rigid behavior.
❑   **a.** Has unusual fears
❑   **b.** Has narrow food preferences
❑   **c.** Carries a specific object
❑   **d** Plays games or completes activities in a repetitive manner or makes own rules for them
❑   **e.** Insists on driving a specific route
❑   **f.** Arranges toys/objects/furniture in a specific way
❑   **g.** Is unable to accept environmental changes (must always go to the same restaurant, same vacation spot)
❑   **h.** Is unable to change the way she has been taught to complete a task
❑   **i.** Needs to be first in line, first selected, etc.
❑   **j.** Erases over and over to make the letters just right
❑   **k.** Colors with so much pressure the crayons break (in order to cover all the white)
❑   **l.** Only sits in one specific chair or one specific location
❑   **m.** Cannot extend the allotted time for an activity; activities must start and end at the times specified
❑   **n.** Selects play choices/interests not commonly shared by others (electricity, weather, advanced computer skills, scores of various sporting events [but not interested in the actual play; this could also be true for music, movies, and books])
❑   **o.** Has narrow clothing preferences
❑   **p.** Feels need to complete projects in one sitting, has difficulty with projects completed over time

C. Failure to follow rules and routines results in behavioral difficulties. These can include:

❑ **1.** Anxiety

❑ **2.** Tantrums/meltdowns (crying, aggression, property destruction, screaming, verbal arguing)

❑ **3.** Noncompliant behaviors

❑ **4.** Increase in perseverative/obsessive/rigid/ritualistic behaviors or preoccupation with area of special interest, engaging in nonsense talk

❑ **5.** Inability to prevent or lessen extreme behavioral reactions, inability to
use coping or calming techniques

❑ **6.** Emotional responses out of proportion to the situation, emotional responses that are more intense and tend to be negative (glass half-empty)

IV. MOTOR CLUMSINESS. THIS REFERS TO DIFFICULTIES WITH MOTOR FUNCTIONING AND PLANNING. THE ASPERGER INDIVIDUAL CAN HAVE DIFFICULTY WITH BOTH GROSS AND FINE MOTOR SKILLS.

A. Difficulties with gross motor skills

❑ **1.** An awkward gait when walking or running

❑ **2.** Poor balance

❑ **3.** Difficulty when throwing or catching a ball (appears afraid of the
ball)

❑ **4.** Difficulty coordinating different extremities, motor planning (shoe tying,
bike riding)

❑ **5.** Difficulty with motor imitation skills

❑ **6.** Difficulty with rhythm copying

❑ **7.** Difficulty with skipping

B. Difficulties with fine motor skills

❑ **1.** Difficulty with handwriting/cutting/coloring skills

❑ **2.** An unusual pencil/pen grasp

❑ **3.** Rushes through fine motor tasks

❑ **4.** Difficulty applying sufficient pressure when writing, drawing, or coloring

❑ **5.** Difficulty with independently seeing sequential steps to complete finished product

❑ **6.** Frustration if writing samples are not perfectly identical to the presented model

V. COGNITIVE ISSUES

A. Mindblindness (theory of mind). This refers to the individual's ability to predict relationships between external and internal states. It is the ability to make inferences about what another person is thinking.

❑ **1.** Is unaware that others have thoughts, beliefs, and desires that influence their behavior

❑ **2.** Views the world in black and white (admits to breaking a rule even when there is no chance of getting caught)

❑ **3.** Is unaware that others have intentions or viewpoints different from her own; when engaging in off-topic conversation, does not realize the listener is having great difficulty following the conversation

❑ **4.** Displays a lack of empathy for others and their emotions (takes another person's belongings)

❑ **5.** Is unaware she can say something that will hurt someone else's feelings or that an apology would make a person feel better (tells another person their story is boring)

❑ **6.** Prefers factual reading materials, rather than fiction

❑ **7.** Has impaired reading comprehension; word recognition is more advanced (difficulty understanding characters in stories, why they do or do not do something)

❑ **8.** Displays difficulty with inferential thinking and problem solving (completing a multistep task that is novel)

B. Lack of cognitive flexibility. This refers to the individual's ability to problem solve, to engage in and maintain mental planning, to exert impulse control, to be flexible in thoughts and actions, and to stay focused on a goal until its completion. Note if there are differences displayed in individual and small and large group settings.

❑ **1.** Is distractable, has difficulty sustaining attention.
❑   **a.** Has difficulty with organizational skills (What do I need to do, and how do I go about implementing it?)
❑   **b.** Has difficulty with sequencing (What is the order used to complete a particular task?)
❑   **c.** Has difficulty with task initiation
❑   **d.** Has difficulty with task completion
❑   **e.** Has difficulty with direction following
❑   **f.** Has difficulty when novel material is presented without visual support
❑   **g.** Engages in competing behaviors (vocalizations, noises, plays with an object, sits incorrectly, looks in wrong direction)

❑ **2.** Has poor impulse control, displays difficulty monitoring own behavior, is not aware of the consequences of her own behavior

❑ **3.** Displays rigidity in thoughts and actions.

- ❑ **a.** Shows a strong desire to control the environment
- ❑ **b.** Has difficulty with transitions
- ❑ **c.** Has difficulty incorporating new information with previously acquired information (information processing, concept formation, analyzing/ synthesizing information), is unable to generalize learning from one situation to another, may behave quite differently in different settings and with different individuals
- ❑ **d.** Engages in repetitive/stereotypic behaviors
- ❑ **e.** Displays a strong need for perfection, wants to complete activities/ assignments perfectly (her standards are very high—noncompliance may stem from avoidance of a task she feels she cannot complete perfectly)

❑ **4.** Displays inflexible thinking, not learning from past mistakes (this is why consequences often appear ineffective)

❑ **5.** Can only focus on one way to solve a problem, though this solution may be ineffective.
- ❑ **a.** Does not ask for help with a problem
- ❑ **b.** Does not ask a peer or adult for needed materials
- ❑ **c.** Continues to engage in an ineffective behavior, rather than thinking of alternatives
- ❑ **d.** Is able to name all the presidents, but not sure what a president does
- ❑ **e.** Is unable to focus on group goals when she is a member of a group

C. **Impaired imaginative play.** This refers to the ability to create and act out novel play scenarios. While the Asperger individual may seem to engage in imaginative play, a closer look reveals play that appears to have an imaginary theme (in terms of characters and topics), but is actually very rigid and repetitive. It is important to observe free play/free time choices. Is the play really novel or is it a retelling of a TV show or video? If the play is novel, can it be changed, can playmates alter it, or is the same play repeated over and over?

❑ **1.** Uses limited play themes and/or toys

❑ **2.** Uses toys in an unusual manner

❑ **3.** Attempts to control all aspects of the play activity; any attempts by others to vary the play are met with firm resistance

❑ **4.** Follows a predetermined script in play

❑ **5.** Engages in play that, although it may seem imaginary in nature, is often a retelling of a favorite movie/TV show/book (this maintains rigidity in thoughts, language, and actions)

❑ **6.** Focuses on special interests such that they dominate play and activity choices

D. Visual learning strength. This refers to being able to learn most successfully through visual modes. This is especially true for the Asperger individual. Visual information remains stable over time, allowing the individual to process, respond, and remember the information (I don't have to worry about forgetting, I can take my time, the information is still there). Not only is this person a visual learner, but she is also a visual thinker. Visual learning compensates for many of the person's areas of need.

❑ **1.** Benefits from schedules, signs, cue cards.
❑   **a.** Uses visual information to help focus attention (I know what to look at)
❑   **b.** Uses visual information as a "backup" (I have something to look at when I forget), especially when new information is presented
❑   **c.** Uses visual information to provide external organization and structure, replacing the individual's lack of internal structure (I know how it is done, I know the sequence)
❑   **d.** Uses visual information to make concepts more concrete
❑   **e.** Uses visual information as a prompt

E. Specific strengths in cognitive areas

❑ **1.** Displays average or above average intellectual ability

❑ **2.** Displays average or above average receptive and expressive language skills

❑ **3.** Has an extensive fund of factual information

❑ **4.** Has an excellent rote memory

❑ **5.** Displays high moral standard (does not know how to lie)

❑ **6.** Displays strong letter recognition skills

❑ **7.** Displays strong number recognition skills

❑ **8.** Displays strong word recognition skills

❑ **9.** Displays strong oral reading skills, though expression and comprehension are limited

❑ **10.** Displays strong spelling skills

VI. SENSORY SENSITIVITIES. THIS REFERS TO ANY ABNORMALITIES OF THE SENSES AN INDIVIDUAL MAY HAVE.

A. Abnormalities in sight, sound, smell, touch, or taste. The Asperger individual generally has difficulty in at least one of these areas, though the degree will vary from person to person. Some individuals may have difficulty in multiple or even all areas. He perceives ordinary sensations as unbearably intense. He will begin to anticipate these experiences, feeling anxious well before the experience occurs. It will be very important to determine if the response is due to sensory or behavioral (learned) difficulties. Often a behavior may initially stem from sensory difficulties, but then become a learned behavior (habit). How you address the behavior will depend on which it is.

❑ **1.** Has difficulty in visual areas.
❑   **a.** Engages in intense staring
❑   **b.** Avoids eye contact

❑   c. Stands too close to objects or people

❑   d. Displays discomfort/anxiety when looking at certain pictures (the individual feels as if the visual experience is closing in on him)

❑ 2. Has difficulty in auditory areas.

❑   a. Covers ears when certain sounds are made

❑   b. Displays extreme fear when unexpected noises occur

❑   c. Displays an inability to focus when surrounded by multiple sounds (shopping mall, airport, party)

❑   d. Purposely withdraws to avoid noises

❑   e. Is fearful of the sounds particular objects make (vacuum, blender, DustBuster)

❑ 3. Has difficulty in olfactory areas.

❑   a. Finds some smells so overpowering or unpleasant that he becomes nauseated

❑   b. Displays a strong olfactory memory

❑   c. Can recognize smells before others

❑   d. Needs to smell foods before eating them

❑   e. Needs to smell materials before using them

❑ 4. Has difficulty in tactile areas.

❑   a. Has difficulty when touched by others, even lightly (especially shoulders and head)

❑   b. Displays anxiety when touched unexpectedly

❑   c. Complains of clothing feeling like sandpaper

❑   d. Has difficulty accepting new clothing (including for change of seasons)

❑   e. Has difficulty with clothing seams or tags

❑   f. Does not respond to temperature appropriately

❑   g. Underreacts to pain

❑   h. Overreacts to pain

❑   i. Has difficulty using particular materials (glue, paint, clay)

❑   j. Complains of a small amount of wetness (from the water fountain, a small spill)

❑ **5.** Has difficulty in gustatory areas.
❑   **a.** Makes limited food choices
❑   **b.** Will only tolerate foods of a particular texture or color
❑   **c.** Needs to touch foods before eating them
❑   **d.** Displays unusual chewing and swallowing behaviors
❑   **e.** Has rigidity issues tied in with limited food preferences (this is the food I always have—it is always this brand and it is always prepared and presented in this way)
❑   **f.** Cannot allow foods to touch each other on the plate
❑   **g.** Must eat each individual food in its entirety before the next
❑   **h.** Has an easily activated gag/vomit reflex

❑ **6.** Engages in self-stimulatory behaviors (rocking, hand movements, facial grimaces)

❑ **7.** Is oversensitive to environmental stimulation (changes in light, sound, smell, location of objects)

❑ **8.** Is undersensitive to environmental stimulation (changes in light, sound, smell, location of objects)

Sohn Grayson Rating Scale for Asperger's Syndrome and High-Functioning Pervasive Developmental Disorder

Student's Name: _____   Evaluator: _____

Birthdate: _____   Date of Evaluation: _____

Diagnosis: _____   Current Placement: _____

SCORE: _____

Below is a list of behaviors. For each item please circle the number that most accurately describes the child's behavior. Please answer all items. When completed, total items in all sections. Higher scores indicate the child or adolescent is displaying more behaviors that may interfere with daily functioning.

1 not true   **2** rarely true   **3** sometimes true   **4** often true

SOCIAL AND BEHAVIORAL

1 2 3 4   1. The child has few preferred friends.

1 2 3 4   2. The child rarely initiates play with others.

1 2 3 4   3. The child rarely engages in imaginative play.

1 2 3 4   4. The child tends to play with particular toys in a repetitive manner.

1　2　3　4　　　　5. The child avoids eye contact.

1　2　3　4　　　　6. The child makes limited use of facial expressions and body language to facilitate communication.

1　2　3　4　　　　7. The child attempts to control play situations (fails to sustain an interest in the play of others).

1　2　3　4　　　　8. The child has difficulty in crowds.

1　2　3　4　　　　9. The child cannot take the perspective of others or understand that others have feelings and thoughts.

1　2　3　4　　　10. The child lacks understanding of others' emotions.

1　2　3　4　　　11. The child has difficulty expressing his or her emotions appropriately.

1　2　3　4　　　12. The child prefers structured activities over nonstructured ones.

1　2　3　4　　　13. The child shows a lack of awareness of others' personal space.

1　2　3　4　　　14. The child has difficulty learning the rules of a game or interaction.

BEHAVIORAL

1　2　3　4　　　　1. The child displays unusual fears.

1　2　3　4　　　　2. The child displays an obsessive interest in narrow or atypical topics (is ritualistic).

1　2　3　4　　　　3. The child is rule bound (sees things in black and white).

1　2　3　4　　　　4. The child displays unusual eating habits.

1　2　3　4　　　　5. The child engages in perseverative behaviors.

1　2　3　4　　　　6. The child's behavior is rigid (has difficulty with changes and transitions, needs sameness, needs order).

1 2 3 4   7. The child is a perfectionist (cannot tolerate mistakes, resists learning new tasks).

1 2 3 4   8. The child appears anxious.

SPEECH AND LANGUAGE

1 2 3 4   1. The child uses words in a peculiar manner.

1 2 3 4   2. The child does not ask for the meaning of words.

1 2 3 4   3. The child does not ask for help.

1 2 3 4   4. The child does not make jokes and has difficulty understanding joking and teasing.

1 2 3 4   5. The child does not initiate conversation.

1 2 3 4   6. The child has difficulty maintaining conversation in a reciprocal format (conversational give-and-take).

1 2 3 4   7. The child does not inquire about others.

1 2 3 4   8. The child "sounds" like an adult.

1 2 3 4   9. The child says things that embarrasses others (comments on physical characteristics, asks probing questions).

1 2 3 4   10. The child engages in obsessive questioning.

1 2 3 4   11. The child engages in obsessive talking about specific topics.

1 2 3 4   12. The child does not maintain another's topic when it does not pertain to his or her own special interest.

1 2 3 4   13. The child has a large vocabulary consisting primarily of nouns and verbs.

1 2 3 4   14. The child does not use language socially (focuses conversations on facts or special interests).

1 2 3 4   15. The child confuses "he" and "she."

1 2 3 4   16. The child displays unusual intonation, pitch, and/or loudness.

1 2 3 4   17. The child uses "language scripts" when conversing (language consists of scripts or parts of scripts from movies/TV/books).

1 2 3 4   18. The child interprets language on a literal level.

1 2 3 4   19. The child misses the point or main idea of a conversation.

1 2 3 4   20. The child insists upon verbal rituals (repeats scripts from movies/TV/books, shares too many details).

1 2 3 4   21. The child does not exhibit gestural communication.

1 2 3 4   22. The child has difficulty maintaining the topic in a conversation.

COGNITION

1 2 3 4   1. The child has difficulty understanding abstract concepts (such as guessing, wishing, time sequence).

1 2 3 4   2. The child displays strong memory skills.

1 2 3 4   3. The child has difficulty with fine motor skills.

1 2 3 4   4. The child interprets the behavior of others on a literal level.

1 2 3 4   5. The child does not generalize learning from one situation to another.

1 2 3 4   6. The child is easily distracted.

1 2 3 4   7. The child has difficulty sustaining attention.

SENSORY

1 2 3 4   1. The child displays unusual sensitivity to noises.

1 2 3 4   2. The child displays unusual sensitivity to smells.

1 2 3 4   3. The child displays unusual sensitivity to tastes.

1 2 3 4   4. The child displays unusual sensitivity to textures.

1 2 3 4   5. The child displays unusual sensitivity to being touched.

1 2 3 4   6. The child engages in repetitive or stereotypic movements.

1 2 3 4   7. The child displays difficulty with motor functioning/ planning (tying shoes, riding a bike).

Rating Scale Results

Score	Probability of Asperger's Syndrome or High-Functioning PDD
58–89	Very Low
90–118	Low
119–149	Mild to Moderate
150–177	Moderate to High
178–207	High to Very High
208–232	Very High

"How to Play a Game"
(Example of a Visual)

1. Pick a game to play:
    _____   _____
    _____   _____
    _____   _____

2. Learn the rules:
    - Where to start
    - Where to end
    - How to move
    - What to touch
    - What to do when you move

3. Ask someone to play:
    - "Would you like to play _____?"
    - "Do you want to play _____?"

4. When you play you must:
    - Follow the game rules
    - Decide who goes first
    - Take turns
    - Ask for help if you don't know how to play
    - Wait your turn
    - Only touch your game piece

- Make nice comments:
  "You can go first."
  "Good try."
  "Don't worry, you'll get another turn."
  "I can show you how to do it."

5. Playing is fun. Sometimes you lose and sometimes you win.
   - Be a good sport—say:
     "Good job."
     "Congratulations!"
     "I had fun."

Problem Wheel
(Example of a Visual)

Problem Wheel

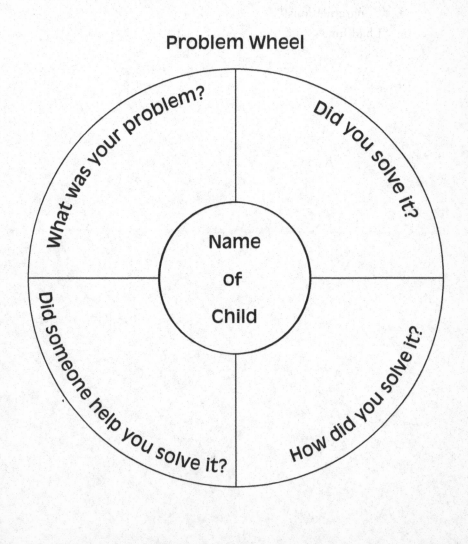

Parent Questionnaire

Name: _____ **Date:** _____

Please complete and return to me as soon as possible. This will help us in getting to know your child. Thank you.

1. By what name do you usually call your child?

2. What are the names and ages of siblings?

3. Is your child currently taking any medications? (If yes, name medications and their dosages.) Does your child have any allergies?

4. Does your child have any health needs or special diet we should know of?

5. What does your child especially dislike? (Give multiple examples.)

6. What does your child especially like? (Give multiple examples.)

7. Does your child have any special fears?

8. Are there any eating habits we should be aware of?

9. Are there any toileting habits we should be aware of?

10. How would you describe your child's sleeping habits?

11. When not involved with a peer or adult, how will your child occupy himself? (Be specific.)

12. Describe your child's social skills with peers (be specific).

13. Please list the names and ages of friends your child may have outside of school.

14. What areas would you most like developed in your child?

15. What are your primary concerns for your child?

Please add any additional information, especially problems you feel would be important for us to know in order to meet your child's needs.

End-of-Year Evaluation

Name: _____ Date: _____

The children have had a productive year. They have learned many new skills, and we have learned through them. As part of this year's review, we would like to have your feelings about the school/home component of our program. Hopefully, through your answers to the following questions, our program will grow and be even more productive next year. Your comments on each question are especially important: try to make specific comments for each question. Thank you.

1. How might our classroom program better meet the needs of your child?

2. Have you seen progress based on the goals outlined in your child's IEP?
   ____ **Yes.** ____ **No.** Comments: (Please mention strength and weakness areas for your child based on the attainment of specific IEP goals.)

3. Are there additional goals you would like to see in your child's IEP next year?
   ____ **Yes.** ____ **No.** Comments:

4. Has your child progressed in areas not mentioned on the IEP?
   ____ **Yes.** ____ **No.** Comments: (Please mention the specific areas where you have seen progress.)

5. What would you like to see added to the classroom program? Please be specific.

6. Were you satisfied with the way you received information (e.g., notes, calls, meetings, etc.)?
_____ **Yes.** _____ **No.** Comments:

7. Do you feel you had enough contact with school and sufficient help in handling problems that arose at home?
_____ **Yes.** _____ **No.** Comments:

8. Do you have needs that have not been met?
_____ **Yes.** _____ **No.** Comments:

9. Do you feel it was a positive and productive school year for your child?
_____ **Yes.** _____ **No.** Comments:

10. Rate the overall classroom program (please circle):
EXCELLENT   GOOD   FAIR   POOR
Comments:

Thank you for taking the time to fill out the evaluation. Your suggestions and comments will help us in planning our program for next year.

Outline for Evaluation Information
for the Asperger Child

The following evaluation format can be used by professionals who wish to create a comprehensive report for children on the Autism spectrum, including those diagnosed with Asperger's syndrome. Most of the items listed here should be evaluated in the assessment of a child on the Autistic spectrum. Not all items, however, will pertain to all children. But it is important that the assessment of your child or teen include more than numerical scores. Look for information on each of these areas in reports from professionals who evaluate your child. Also look for their explanations of each concept.

I. BACKGROUND INFORMATION

A. Birth and Early Development

B. Previous Evaluations
1. Educational
2. Medical
3. Other

C. School History

D. Medical History
1. Hearing
2. Vision
3. Medications

II. CURRENT FUNCTIONING (HOME VS. SCHOOL/OBSERVED VS. REPORTED)

A. Test Results

B. Cognitive Functioning
   1. Cause-and-effect understanding
   2. Object functioning
   3. Creative play
   4. Concrete vs. abstract thinking
   5. Generalization of skills
   6. Memory skills
   7. Object relations
   8. Intellectual functioning

C. Communication Skills
   1. Receptive language
   2. Expressive language
   3. Communicative intent
   4. Mode of communication
      a. Nonverbal (nonspecific): crying, gestures, pulling other person, grabbing, noises, head shakes
      b. Nonverbal (specific): signing, picture exchange, assistive devices
      c. Verbal: one, two, three words; phrases; sentences
      d. Echolalia
      e. Perseveration
      f. Stereotypical phrases/dialogue
      g. Quality (tone, pitch, speed, etc.)

D. Rate and Sequence of Development
   1. Splinter skills
   2. Skill regression
   3. Evenness of skills

E. Social Interactions
   1. Relationships with others: adults, peers, family

2. Eye contact
3. In structured activities
4. At play time

F. **Sensory Issues**
   1. Visual
      a. Staring responses
      b. Distractibility
      c. Withdrawal
      d. Self-stimulation
   2. Auditory
      a. Localization
      b. Response to name
      c. Selective attention
      d. Distractibility
      e. Withdrawal
      f. Self-stimulation
   3. Tactile/kinesthetic
      a. Self-stimulation
      b. Defensiveness
      c. Grimaces or gestures
      d. Degree of activity
      e. Physical responsiveness
      f. Pain response
   4. Olfactory/gustatory
      a. Smelling of objects
      b. Preferences and aversions to foods and/or textures
      c. Mouthing objects

G. **Behaviors**
   1. Functional assessment of behaviors:
        Behavior   Antecedents   Consequences
   2. Motivational assessment scale
   3. Other issues:
      a. Repetitive, stereotyped, or ritualistic behaviors

    b. Resistance to change

    c. Fears and anxieties

    d. Affect

    e. Aggression

    f. Self-injurious behaviors

    g. Tantrums

    h. Elopement

    i. Response to demands

    j. Frustration responses

    k. Transitioning

    l. Compliance

H. Prerequisite Learning Behaviors

    1. Sitting in a chair to work

    2. On-task time

    3. Eye contact

    4. Attention to task

    5. Degree of independence: performs skill with physical prompt, modeling prompt, verbal prompt, independently and/or spontaneously with supervision, independently in a practical way

I. Motor Functioning: Fine and Gross

J. Self-Help Skills

    1. Grooming

    2. Eating/drinking

    3. Toileting

    4. Dressing

K. Academic Skills

Recommended Social Skills Materials

Begun, Ruth, ed. 1995. *Ready-to-Use Social Skills Lessons and Activities for Grades PreK–K*. West Nyack, NY: Center for Applied Research in Education.

Gajewski, Nancy, Polly Hirn, and Patty Mayo. 1993–1996. *Social Star: Books 1 to 3*. Eau Claire, WI: Thinking Publications.

Gray, Carol. Various books and videotapes, available through Future Horizons, www.futurehorizons-autism.com or (800) 489-0727.

Mannix, Darlene. 1992. *Life Skills Activities for Special Children*. West Nyack, NY: Center for Applied Research in Education.

———. 1993. *Social Skills Activities for Special Children*. West Nyack, NY: Center for Applied Research in Education.

Wilson, Carolyn C. *Room 14: A Social Language Program*. East Moline, IL: LinguiSystems. Available at www.linguisystems.com or (800) 776-4332.

Winner, Michelle Garcia. 2000. *Inside Out: What Makes the Person with Social Cognitive Deficits Tick?* Available at www.socialthinking.com or (408) 557-8595.

———. 2002. *Thinking about You Thinking about Me*. Available at www.social thinking.com or (408) 557-8595.

INDEX

Activities
  flexibility and, 149
  preferred v. nonpreferred, 32–33
  scheduling and, 86–87
ADHD. *See* Attention Deficit Hyperactivity
    Disorder
Alice in Wonderland, 227
American Psychiatric Association, 1
Angry/resistant boy
  characteristics of, 60
  recommended approach for, 60–61
Anxiety
  Asperger individuals and, 2, 33–34
  causes of, 33
  control and, 118, 177
  coping strategies for, 60
  crisis and, 175
  environmental controls and, 68–69
  guide and, 70
  intervention strategies for, 16
  management of, 123–25
  manifestations of, 34, 35
  obsessive-compulsive issues and, 33–34
  perfectionism and, 216–17
  prevention of, 16
  recognition of, 33
  rigidity and, 141
  routines, schedules and, 4, 86
  sabotage and, 144–45
  social interactions and, 38, 154
  social rules and, 15–16
  societal rules and, 30–31
  sources of, 124
  of students, 212–13
Anxiety boy

  characteristics of, 58–59
  recommended approach to, 59–60
Asperger, Hans, 1
Asperger individuals. *See also* Teenagers
  anxiety in, 2, 33–34
  behavior change of, 14
  behavioral function of, 28
  black-and-white thinking of, 34, 36, 39
  cognitive restructuring for, 181–82
  coping skills for, 42, 49
  differences in, 48–49
  discussion with, 104–6
  distress of, 40
  Emotion boy as, 54
  emotional issues for, 96–97
  energy conservation of, 38–39
  fitting in and, 10–11
  forced choices for, 111–16
  frames of reference for, 31–32
  help for, 5–6
  internalizers v. externalizers and, 40–41
  language for, 39–40
  Logic boy as, 51–54
  middle ground for, 106–9
  new thinking for, 103–4
  perfectionism of, 39
  preferred v. nonpreferred activities for,
    32–33
  preventive strategies and, 63–64
  problem prevention and, 65, 67–68
  problem solving of, 14–15
  progress, improvement for, 198
  pushing of, 199–200
  rehearsals, role-playing for, 110–11
  reinforcers for, 69–70

Asperger individuals: *(cont)*
    replacement skills for, 44
    rigidity of, 31
    Rule boy as, 49–51
    self-calming by, 125–35
    sexual issues for, 95–96
    social intelligence and, 153–54
    social interactions for, 162
    social skills and, 151, 154, 155–64
    societal rules and, 30–31
    special interests of, 149
    strategies for, 19–20
    structure for, 20–21
    success for, 202–3
    teacher interaction with, 208–9
    teaching to, 205–27
    thriving of, 137
    visuals for, 84–93
Asperger students
    academic needs of, 215–16
    anxiety reduction for, 212–13
    assessment of, 209–10
    attention of, 217–18
    blending in and, 217
    change, challenges for, 205–6
    contingency accommodations for, 224–26
    environment for, 211
    inclusion of, 223–26
    language with, 213–15
    mainstreaming of, 219–23
    needs of, 207–8
    observation of, 210
    perfectionism and, 216–17
    prevention, sabotage for, 218–19
    reward system for, 217–18
    skill-centered intervention for, 211, 213
    subtypes and, 210
    support for, 222–23
    teachers, parents and, 227
Asperger's syndrome
    ADHD and, 38, 55
    anxiety and, 2, 33–34, 123–25
    Anxiety Boy subtype of, 58–60
    approach to, 14
    assessment of, 259–62
    behavioral function and, 28
    characteristics checklist for, 229–46
    characteristics of, 1–2, 3–5
    clumsiness and, 4
    cognitive issues of, 4–5
    cognitive skills of, 3, 240–44
    crisis intervention and, 175–96

    crisis situations and, 23–24
    depression and, 201
    diagnosis of, 1, 11–15
    fantasy subtype and, 57–58
    features of, 12
    flexibility and, 2
    future planning and, 199–200
    generalization, sabotage and, 21–23
    individuality of, 229
    instruments for, 9
    interpretation and, 1–2
    language skills and, 3–4, 6, 234–37
    medication and, 54, 201–2
    mindblindness and, 4–5, 36
    motor functioning and, 239–40
    OCD and, 55–56
    prevention and, 6
    professionals for, 198
    rigidity of, 29
    rituals and, 9–10, 12
    routines and, 4, 237–39
    school and, 41–43
    sensory sensitivities and, 5, 38
    social interactions and, 3, 12, 36–38,
        94–95, 230–34
    social skills and, 151
    social stories and, 10
    sphere of influence for, 21
    structure, predictability and, 20–21
    subtypes of, 20, 47–62
Attention Deficit Hyperactivity Disorder
    (ADHD), 11, 29
    Asperger's syndrome and, 55
    description of, 56
    issues of, 38
    medication for, 201
    recommendations for, 56
Autistic spectrum disorders, 13

Behavior
    analysis of, 65
    anxiety and, 33–34, 35
    black-and-white thinking and, 34, 36
    frames of reference for, 31–32
    function of, 18–19, 28
    important issues and, 36–43
    issues of, 163–64
    motivations for, 18
    obsessive-compulsive, 106
    preferred v. nonpreferred activities and,
        32–33
    reasons for, 17–19, 27–45, 37, 229

replacement, 118
social interactions and, 36–38
societal rules and, 30–31
triggers of, 43–45
Body language
social interactions and, 233–34
social skill development and, 167

Checklists
of cognitive skills, 240–44
of interests, routines, 237–39
of language skills, 234–37
of motor functioning, planning, 239–40
for sensory sensitivities, 244–46
of social interactions, 230–34
use of, 89–90
Classroom
consistency and, 205
guidelines for, 211
learners in, 206–7
prevention strategies in, 218–19
Cognitive skills
black-and-white thinking and, 34, 36
checklist of, 240–44
flexibility of, 241–42
imaginative play and, 242–43
mindblindness and, 4–5, 36
strengths in, 243–44
visual learning and, 243
Cognitive Social Integration Therapy (CSIT), 6
anxiety and, 16
behavioral function and, 17–19
core components of, 17–25
crisis situations and, 23–24, 175
description of, 15–16
effectiveness of, 139
final goal of, 24–25
generalization, sabotage and, 21–23
goal of, 64
instruction and, 17
planned sabotage and, 144
in school setting, 207
social component of, 6–7
sphere of influence and, 21
structure, predictability and, 20–21
subtypes and, 19–20
techniques for, 139
use of, 15, 16–17
Communication
social skills development and, 165–66
Control
anxiety and, 177

consequences to, 116
in environment, 68
forced choices and, 112, 116
by parents, 100–101
of speaking volume, 92–93
teaching of, 100–102
Conversation
parts of, 170
scripts for, 72–73, 166
skills for, 166
social skill development and, 166–67
topics for, 170
types of, 167
Coping skills
stress resiliency and, 120
teaching of, 119–20
Crisis
being okay in, 134
control in, 177
flexibility and, 178
goals in, 175
planning for, 194–96
Crisis intervention, 175–96
calming child and, 180–81
child's understanding and, 185
choices and, 181
compliance task and, 181
frustration, challenges, changes and, 186–87
good choice/bad choice technique for, 187–88
labeling problem in, 181
planning and, 194–96
private place for, 180
problems, solutions technique for, 178, 180–87
role-playing, practice and, 185–86
social stories and, 188–94
solving problem in, 181–84
steps for, 184–87
strategies for, 178–94
ten commandments of, 179
verbal compliance and, 184–85
CSIT. See Cognitive Social Integration Therapy
Cue cards
as visuals, 89

Depression, 201
Diagnosis
difficulties of, 11–15
requirements of, 13

Discussion
  middle ground in, 106–9
  new thinking and, 104–6
  real world and, 106
  visual image for, 104–5

Emotion boy
  angry/resistant subtype of, 60–61
  anxiety boy subtype of, 58–59
  characteristics of, 54
  fantasy boy subtype of, 57–58
  medication for, 54
  negative subtype of, 61
Emotions
  anxiety management and, 123–25
  primary v. secondary, 123
  regulation of, 123
  self-calming and, 125–35
Employment
  Asperger teens and, 97–98
Environment
  control in, 68
  interpersonal, 69
  physical, 68–69
Evaluation
  end-of-year, 257–58
  outline for, 259–62

Fantasy boy
  characteristics of, 57–58
  crisis intervention and, 177–78
  recommended approach to, 58
Fantasy world
  real world v., 106
Flexibility
  compliance and, 149
  crisis intervention and, 178
  generalization and, 142
  hierarchy of change and, 83
  introduction of, 82
  life lessons and, 121
  need for, 138
  overcoming fears and, 148
  through sabotage, 147–50
  social story and, 148, 193
  special interests and, 149
  steps for, 150
  teaching of, 83–84
  transitions and, 84, 149
  for young children, 147
Forced choice
  being okay and, 115
  control and, 112, 116

introduction of, 112
obsessive-compulsive behaviors and, 112–14
teaching of, 111–16

Generalization
  help with, 140–41
  parents and, 227
  phrases for, 141, 142
  practice for, 142–43
  sabotage and, 146
  of skill, 139
  of social skills, 156–57, 161–62
  teaching of, 141–43
Goals
  intervention levels and, 66–67
  selection, prioritization of, 65–67
Gray, Carol, 188, 189

Hand signals
  visuals and, 89

IEP. See Individualized Education Program
Inclusion
  case manager and, 224
  techniques for, 223–26
Individualized Education Program (IEP), 224
  contingency accommodations and, 224–26
Innocent/passive boy
  approach to, 50
  as Rule boy subtype, 49–50
Interventions. See also Prevention strategies
  reframing and, 74–76
  techniques for, 20

Language
  clear, simple, 81–82
  compliance and, 71–74
  conversational scripts and, 72–73, 81
  discussion and, 104
  flexibility and, 83
  generalization, sabotage and, 21–23
  of good choice/bad choice technique, 187
  impairments in, 3–4, 234–37
  issues of, 39–40
  key words, phrases for, 76–84
  pragmatic use of, 154, 234–35
  processing of, 236–37
  prosody and, 4, 236
  reframing and, 74–76
  semantic use of, 235–36
  skills checklist for, 234–37
  specialized needs and, 213–15
  vocal tone, facial expressions and, 80

Learned optimism, 121–22
Learning. *See also* Teaching
  stability for, 64–65
Life lessons, 120–21
Logic boy
  characteristics of, 51–52
  recommended approach to, 52
  social skills and, 152–53

Mainstreaming
  supervised, 220
  teacher modifications and, 221–22
  techniques for, 219–23
  unsupervised, 220–23
Medication
  ADHD and, 201
  teenagers and, 97
Mindblindness, 4–5, 36. *See also* Theory of
    mind
  assessment of, 240–41
Motor skills
  assessment of, 239–40
  difficulty with, 4

Negative boy
  characteristics of, 61
  recommended approach to, 61

Obsessive-Compulsive Disorder (OCD), 11
  Asperger's syndrome and, 55–56
  characteristics of, 56–57
  forced choices and, 111, 112
  recommended approach to, 57
OCD. *See* Obsessive-Compulsive Disorder
Oppositional Defiant Disorder (ODD),
    29, 60
Overcontrolled boy
  as Rule Boy subtype, 51

Paranoid boy
  as Emotion Boy subtype, 54–55
  recommended approach to, 55
Parents
  as child's advocate, expert, 99, 197
  control by, 100–101
  daily life and, 200–201
  as "defender of reality," 158
  demands by, 200
  evaluation by, 198
  generalization and, 227
  as problem solvers, 186
  pushing by, 199–200
  questionnaire for, 255–56

  role of, 197–201
  school involvement and, 226–27
  as "sphere of influence," 100
  teachers and, 227
Peers
  play initiation with, 172–73
  as role models, 163
Perfectionism
  of Asperger student, 216–17
Personal space
  teaching of, 171–72
Perspective-taking
  social situations and, 153–54
Play
  initiation of, 172–73
  skills for, 155–56
Prevention strategies. *See also* Interventions
  behavior analysis and, 65
  in classroom, 218–19
  conversational scripts as, 72–73, 81
  cue cards as, 89
  daily routine as, 70–71
  environmental controls and, 68–69
  flexibility and, 82
  goal selection and, 65–67
  hand signals as, 89
  intervention levels with, 66
  key words, phrases and, 76–84
  language and, 71–74
  reaction v., 67–68
  reframing and, 74–76
  reinforcers and, 69–70
  schedules and, 86–88
  sequence cards, checklists and, 89–92
  step-by-step approach to, 65
  teenagers and, 93
  use of, 63–64
  visuals as, 84–86
  for volume control, 92–93
Problem solving
  "after the fact," 183–84
  steps to, 184
Problems
  being okay with, 126
  frustration, challenges, changes as,
    186–87
  identification of, 81
  manifestations of, 229
  prevention of, 63–64, 67–68, 126
  reframing of, 128
  skills for, 81
Professionals
  evaluation of, 198

Rating scale
  Sohn Grayson, 247–51
Reframing
  of new situations, 74–76
Rigidity
  anxiety and, 141
  assessment of, 237–39
  obsessions and, 106–7, 237–38
  perfectionism and, 216–17
  reasons for, 29
  rules and, 237
  successive approximations and, 134
Role-playing, 110–11
  for crisis intervention, 185–86
  for social skills training, 159–60, 161
Routines
  behavioral difficulties and, 238–39
  insistence on, 237–39
Rule boy
  as Asperger subtype, 48
  characteristics of, 49
  innocent/passive boy and, 49–50
  overcontrolled boy and, 51
  subtypes of, 49

Sabotage
  change and, 147
  choice and, 146–47
  in classroom, 218–19
  flexibility through, 147–50
  generalization and, 146
  importance of, 205–6
  as learning tool, 139
  planning for, 144–47
  times for, 145
  use of, 143–44
Schedule
  development of, 87
  as prevention strategy, 86–88
  sample of, 87–88
School
  environment in, 210
  evaluation from, 227
  "hidden curriculum" of, 42
  high school issues and, 42–43
  inclusion techniques for, 223–26
  mainstreaming in, 219–23
  middle school issues and, 41–42
  parental involvement in, 226–27
  social skills goals for, 165–69
  social skills training and, 157–58
  teasing in, 42
  understanding for, 41

School programs
  academic needs in, 215–16
  anxiety reduction in, 212–13
  assessment and, 209–10
  blending in and, 217
  essentials for, 206–19
  interventions in, 207, 211, 213
  language guidelines for, 214–15
  perfectionism in, 216–17
  reward system in, 217–18
  teaching guidelines for, 208–9
  techniques for, 207
Scripts
  for problem prevention, 72–73, 81
Self-calming, 125–35
  adding visual for, 133
  being okay and, 125–31
  continuation phase to, 134–35
  crisis intervention and, 134
  expanding concept of, 131–32
  individualized approach to, 129–31
  introduction of, 126–31
  obstacles to, 127
  phrases for, 132–33
  props for, 133
  successive approximations for, 134
Sensory development
  checklist for, 244–46
  issues of, 5
Sequence cards
  use of, 89–92
Sex
  teenagers and, 95–96
Sharing
  teaching of, 171
Skills
  generalization of, 139
  learning of, 139
  sabotage and, 139
Social debriefing, 116–18
Social intelligence
  difficulty with, 153–54
Social interactions
  appropriate behaviors and, 233
  of Asperger children, 15
  behavioral issues and, 163–64
  checklist for, 230–34
  desire for, 231–32
  difficulty with, 3, 230–34
  initiating contact and, 94–95
  interest in, 36–38
  keeping current and, 162–63
  nonverbal communication and, 233–34

peers and, 163
preparation for, 18, 19
reciprocal interactions and, 230–31
scheduling of, 162
scripts for, 163–64
social cues and, 232
social debriefing and, 116–18
teenagers and, 94–95
Social skills
  abstract skills and, 168–69
  body language and, 167
  challenge of, 173–74
  change in, 154
  communication and, 165–66
  conversations and, 166–67, 170
  core curriculum for, 165–69
  CSIT and, 7
  development of, 151–74, 155–64
  eye contact and, 169
  fitting in and, 157–58
  generalization of, 161–62
  "good sport" skills and, 167–68
  group participation and, 167
  guidelines for, 155, 158
  initial interactions and, 161
  interaction skills and, 168
  materials for, 169–70
  outside home, 156–57
  personal space and, 169, 171–72
  play initiation and, 172–73
  play skills and, 155
  playmates and, 155–56
  practice for, 160
  recommended materials for, 263
  reward of, 174
  role-playing and, 159–60, 161
  school and, 157–58
  sharing and, 171
  social stories and, 169
  social thinking and, 154
  strategies for, 170–71
  techniques for, 158–59
  training of, 154
  turn taking and, 170
  visuals and, 159
  voice volume and, 170
Social stories, 10
  for being okay, 133
  choices and, 190–91
  development of, 189–90
  flexibility and, 148, 193
  goal of, 193–94
  guidelines for, 189

review of, 191
sample of, 194
social skills development and, 169
technique of, 188–94
use of, 191–92
writing of, 192–94
Social thinking, 154
Sohn Grayson Rating Scale for Asperger's
    Syndrome and High-Functioning
    Pervasive Developmental Disorder,
    247–51
Stress immunity
  life lessons and, 120–21
Stress management
  teaching of, 119–20
Stress resiliency
  teaching of, 120
Structure
  for Asperger child, 20–21
Students. See also Asperger students
  change, challenges for, 205–6

Talking wheel
  volume control and, 92–93
Teachers
  assessment by, 209–10
  behavior style of, 208
  crisis intervention and, 182–83
  guidelines for, 208–9
  modifications for, 221–22
  parents and, 227
  prevention, sabotage and, 218–19
  as problem solvers, 182–83
  receptiveness of, 226
  social stories for, 189, 191–92
Teaching
  academic needs and, 215–16
  anxiety management and, 123–25, 212–13
  of Asperger students, 205–27
  changing course and, 109
  control and, 100–102
  of coping skills, 119–20
  discussion and, 104–6
  emotional regulation and, 123
  environment for, 211
  forced choices and, 111–16
  of generalization, 141–43
  language needs and, 213–15
  of learned optimism, 121–22
  mainstreaming and, 219–23
  of middle-ground, 106–9
  of new skills, 118–19
  new thinking and, 103–4

Teaching: *(cont)*
   of personal space, 171–72
   of real world, 106
   rehearsals, role-playing as, 110–11
   of self-calming, 125–35
   of sharing, 171
   skill-centered interventions and, 211, 213
   social debriefing and, 116–18
   of social skills, 155–64
   "sphere of influence" and, 100
   of stress immunity, 120–21
   of stress management, 119–20
   stress resiliency and, 120
   techniques for, 100
   teens and, 102–3
Teenagers. *See also* Asperger individuals
   emotional issues for, 96–97
   medication issues for, 97
   sexual issues for, 95–96
   social issues for, 94–95
   special considerations for, 93
   teaching of, 102–3

   work and, 97–98
Theory of mind. *See also* Mindblindness
   learning of, 122–23
   social situations and, 153–54
Thinking
   changing of, 103–4

Visuals
   cue cards as, 89
   discussion and, 104–5
   example of, 252–53, 254
   as prevention strategy, 84–85
   for problem solving, 186
   schedules as, 86–88
   sequence cards, checklists and, 89–92
   social skills training and, 159
   talking wheel, volume control and, 92–93
   use of, 84–86
Volume control
   visuals for, 92–93

Work. *See* Employment

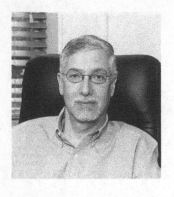

Alan Sohn, Ed.D., has worked with those within the Autistic Spectrum for over twenty years. First, within public schools and then in his own private psychology practice, Dr. Sohn has worked with all ages, from preschoolers to adults. After leaving public schools, his private practice rapidly expanded, and now includes consultation services to a number of school districts and agencies as well as social skills groups for individuals from five to eighteen years of age. In addition, he frequently provides expert testimony in proceedings regarding Autistic Spectrum Disorder. Along with Ms. Grayson he conducts numerous training seminars for both parents and professionals

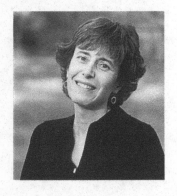

Cathy Grayson, M.A., has worked with children in the Autistic Spectrum in public schools for over twenty-five years. Due to the rising demand for experts in the field of Asperger Syndrome, she has retired from teaching to devote herself to a private consulting practice. Using the techniques outlined in this book Ms. Grayson works with Asperger's children, adolescents, and their families. In addition, she consults with both public and private schools and provides staff training and supervision for their Autistic Spectrum programs. She also offers social skills groups for young children with Asperger Syndrome. Ms. Grayson is an instructor in the education department of LaSalle University where she shares her knowledge and techniques with future teachers.

As the founders of Sohn Grayson Autism Consultants Alan Sohn, Ed.D., and Cathy Grayson, M.A., developed Cognitive Social Integration Therapy (CSIT), an approach that recognizes that the lack of social understanding is the primary difficulty for those with Asperger Syndrome. Their belief is this approach and their own success in using it provided the impetus for this book.